FIVE MIRRORS, FIVE BLESSINGS

Susana Stoica, Ph.D.

The book is an imaginary story and similarities with any person living or dead is merely coincidental.

The content of this book is copyrighted and should not be copied either verbatim or in theory without prior permission from the author.

ISBN-13: 978-1-7322429-7-5

Healing Alternatives Press

Other books by the same author:

Reluctant Healer: An Introduction to Energy Healing

Heal your Brain, Reclaim your Life: How to Recover
and Thrive after a Concussion

Cooking after Brain Injury: Easy Cooking for
Recovery

Healing with the Loving Heart

Those we love most are the ones who can inflict the worst pain on us, but if we took the time to look closer, we would find that they are our best teachers, guiding us on a path of becoming kinder, better, more compassionate individuals.

Susana Stoica

Contents

Introduction
ᖇᕐᕐᕐ

The story of Cassie is a composite of the many people I worked with over the years[1] as well as my own life. I tried to fit as much information as I could into Cassie's profile so you, my reader, can get the maximum possible benefit from her story. I defined Cassie as being in her seventies, so she can claim a lot of different life experiences, and because, unless there is an obvious trauma in their lives - like losing a loved one, people typically tend to work on their emotional traumas later in life. I also defined her as having many aspects to her life, so people can identify at least with some of them. She is a daughter, a sibling, a wife, a mother, and a professional, as all these sides of one's life can provide traumas. I defined her as a busy person, who likes doing things well, and who is fully engaged in all the aspects of her life, a person who would say she wishes she had a "thirty-six-hour day". I made her a "normal" human being, one who did not have excessively cruel trauma inflicted on her so the reader, be it a man or a woman, can relate to her.

---

[1] While I am a Certified Hypnotherapist, as a healer, I can access and remove the trauma patterns directly from a person's energy field, which is a much faster and easier process.

In today's world, people are asked to work increasingly longer hours, then seamlessly switch to taking care of all aspects of one's family's needs. While more men help their wives with home chores, typically the wife would have to take care of most of them, hence my subject is a woman.

I know from my own life experience that the see-saw of "properly" taking care of one's family and being successful in one's profession can be daunting, and one can end up with feelings of failure and inadequacy, especially if one does not have a supporting environment.

This is the story of how, under the guidance of a skilled therapist, a professional woman in her seventies is finally able to make sense of her life experiences.

Meeting My Therapist
ৎৡৡ৶

"Hello! It is nice finally meeting you." the therapist greeted me cheerfully as I entered her office. "I heard so much about you, I feel as if I have known you forever. I was really intrigued by your idea of examining your life. Not many people do it. By the way, you can call me Isabelle. It might make you feel more comfortable. I expect by the end of our work together I will know more about you than anyone else in your life, so you will no longer see me as a stranger." Isabelle winked while showing me to the comfortable sofa in her office.

Isabelle McCowan came highly recommended by a friend who was helped by her. I heard Isabelle was compassionate, a good listener, and patient. The latter was very important for me as, having a tendency of getting lost in details, I knew I needed somebody who does not get impatient, instead can gently bring me back to the subject at hand.

"So, tell me Cassie, where would you like to start, what is most important for you to figure out?" she continued. "Do you have any preference?"

"All I can tell you is that I would like to make sense of all aspects of my life. Looking back at my life, it feels like a basement full of unsorted memorabilia thrown around without any rhyme or reason. I would like to understand why some things happened in my life. I used to beat myself up for not doing enough, and I still do, while people around me were marveling at how I could do so much. Some people praise me while others pass judgment on me for the same events. I want to understand who I really am, warts and all." I said smiling.

"Interesting idea. I would suggest we figure out first how do you perceive your life and match a method of therapy that works with what you want to accomplish. You told me you are into meditation. Is that right?"

"Yes, I am a long-time meditator, and I did quite a bit of work with my past and my emotions, which should make our work easier."

"Yes, all that should help, as I hope you will be able to access the information you need easier than the average person" said Isabelle comfortably settling into her chair. "Do you need some water or coffee before we start?"

"No, thank you. I am ready for our trip together." And with that I settled on the comfortable sofa.

"How do you view your life? What is your general feeling about it? We should find a way to simplify our job by partitioning it. Would that work for you?"

"Yes", I replied readily, "that is exactly what I wanted to suggest. There are two overriding feelings about my life: one of abandonment and a constant stress because of a need to be perfect, to do even more, so I could meet the requirements of being a good, reliable person.

I always felt like I lived my life on several distinct tracks that sometimes interacted, but mostly were self-contained. I had to be perfect in each one of those parts of my life, otherwise I would disappoint my parents, my boss, my husband, my sister. Most of the time I had no idea what the requirements for being 'perfect' were, so I learned to strive to be better and better at what I was doing. While this was stressful, it also made me a good professional and a compassionate, helpful human being."

"Can you tell me more about it?" enquired Isabelle, leaning forward in her chair.

"Yes, as far as I could determine, my main tracks are being a daughter, a sister, a wife, a mother, and a professional."

"Okay, it sounds like you put quite a bit of thinking into this and you already figured out a good way to partition your experiences. I suggest, given your background in meditation, to work with light hypnosis[2], if you feel comfortable with it."

"Yes, I do! I love the easy access it provides to memories."

"So, tell me, which aspect of your life would you like to begin with?"

"What about we do it in a chronological order, examining each track as it entered my life?"

"It is as good an approach as any!" replied Isabelle.

---

[2] When using light hypnosis, a person is completely aware and remembers everything that is being said during a session, while working in a deeply relaxed state, which allows for easy information retrieval.

Being a Daughter
ⓒⓈⓑⓞ

"Please close your eyes and take a few deep breaths. Feel yourself relaxing your whole body head to toe" started Isabelle.

It was easy for me to relax. I fully trusted my therapist, so my old habit of instantaneously relaxing after a few deep breaths kicked in.

"Now imagine yourself in a beautiful garden. It has lush green trees and under the trees you can see colorful flowers. You can even hear birds happily chirping as you walk through this enchanted garden. Enjoy this garden while relaxing more and more as you walk through it. At some point you will see a gazebo. Can you see it?" Isabelle paused waiting for my reply.

"Yes, I can see the garden and the gazebo. I am just going up the steps leading to the gazebo platform."

"You are ahead of me! Can you see inside the gazebo the five body-length mirrors?"

"I can see them clearly. They have ornate frames, such as those in Middle Ages."

"Now imagine a plaque with some lettering on top of each of the mirrors. The plaque on the first mirror lists 'Being a Daughter', the next 'Being a Sister', then 'Being a Wife', followed by 'Being a Mother', and 'Being a Professional'."

"Yes, I can clearly read the plaques. The lettering is golden and ornate."

"Don't focus on the lettering, just know it is there. Now, imagine that each of these mirrors is in fact an access door to the specific memories labeled above them. Can you do that?"

"Yes, no problem. This is shaping up to be a real adventure. Can we go through the 'Being a Daughter' one?"

"Yes. Just step through the mirror. As soon as you step through, you find yourself looking at your parents just before you were born. What do you see?"

"My parents are very much in love. They are Holocaust survivors and having me is like building again what they lost in the war: a family. I can see my aunt in the house. She is so young. She came back from Auschwitz barely alive and my mom is doting on her. My father is the practical one. He wants my aunt to go fulfill her prewar dream of being a doctor, but my aunt just wants to live, make up for the time she lost when at only fifteen she was taken to the concentration camp.

Next I see my mom in her late pregnancy. My dad had to go to another city, to obtain his engineering diploma. He began his studies before the war in Romania. He survived the *numerus clausus*[3] but, being born in Transylvania, when Romania ceded Transylvania to Hungary in 1940, he had to return home and chose to continue his studies in Brno, Czechoslovakia. He had to flee from there too when the Nazis entered the city. After that, he decided to continue his studies in Budapest, Hungary. That is where the Nazis caught up with him and he was sent to a forced labor camp in Wiener Neustadt. He survived because he was fluent in German and had the ability to repair just about anything.

After the war, with the parents perished in the Holocaust, my father became head of the family, taking care of both his and my mom's sister for a while.

---

[3] **Numerus clausus** ("closed number" in Latin) is one of many methods used to limit the number of students who may study at a university. In many cases, the goal of the *numerus clausus* was simply to limit the number of students to the maximum feasible in some particularly sought-after areas of studies. However, in some cases, *numerus clausus* policies were religious or racial quotas, both in intent and function. (from Wikipedia.com) With the rise of Nazi Germany, Romanian universities introduced a 5% quota for Jewish students.

He knew he needed to finish his studies in order to be able to provide for his family.

By an unbelievable stroke of luck, my father was able to find his exam records in the rubble of the Budapest University and, as such, had the necessary documents to finish his studies where he originally began: in Romania, at the Bucharest Polytechnic Institute. He finished his studies *Summa Cum Laude*[4] just in the nick of time, merely days before I was born. I was one of the first Jewish children in our city, Târgu-Mureș [*Marosvásárhely* in Hungarian] and as such my mom was celebrated by the whole community as a symbol of survival. It wasn't easy though. My mother had problems bonding with me, something that was not unusual for women who lost their families in the Holocaust. There were also great food shortages. Luckily my father was assigned to a group of people who drove heavy trucks to Czechoslovakia to bring tooling for factories. It seems that in Czechoslovakia people had more food, so my dad was able to bring some for us too.

I see my mother working hard to take care of me and her sister. All I can see is mom cooking in the kitchen.

Both mom and dad suffered terribly because of losing their parents in Auschwitz. After I started kindergarten, the usual morning scene was my father

---

[4] *Summa Cum Laude* [Latin] – with distinction

brushing my hair and braiding it while telling me stories about his mother, who had beautiful long hair, my grandfather who loved and respected her very much, and his two brothers who perished in Transnistria forced labor camp. My mom was so affected by the Holocaust, she rarely talked about her side of the family. I remember that for me it did not make any sense. How could my dad, who was a parent, a grownup, have himself parents? Only later did I realize that I was missing something: I was missing having grandparents! I realized that only when I went to school and my classmates told me with joy that they were going to spend their summer at their grandparents' house.

When I was about five, my father was sent to Bucharest[5], to work in planning the postwar Romanian economy. Engineers, especially good ones, were at a premium at the time, as the communist regime did not trust the intellectuals who got their diplomas before the war[6].

Eventually my mother joined my dad and I was left behind with my aunt, who at that time was studying

---

[5] Bucharest [*Bucureşti* in Romanian] is the capital city of Romania.
[6] It would take many years and a serious review of the person's war time history before somebody would be allowed to teach or have any important position related to the redevelopment of the Romanian economy after the war. The communists were very afraid of sabotage.

to become a pediatrician. My aunt, Julia, was very kind and loving. She was more like a big sister to me than an aunt, as she was practically raised by my parents. She told me years later about my mom's problems related to bonding with me and the fact that once I was left behind, in Târgu-Mureș by my parents, my mom was not eager to have me again. Before my parents finally took me with them, my aunt Julia had to repeatedly complain to my parents that she would fail her exams unless they took me back.

I found out about the above only because I asked Julia if she had any clue about my deep feeling of abandonment that I could not figure out. I was in my sixties at the time.

I can see myself during my time with my aunt being taken by her and her future husband on their dates. They told me they loved buying me a certain magazine because I happily 'read' it while in the stroller and it looked very funny. As soon as I could eat it, they always bought me fresh popcorn made by vendors on the street. I always felt very safe with them and I was grateful for their love. In fact, my sweetest childhood memories are related to them and their children.

When I was about five I realized, at an intuitive level, that my parents harbored much sorrow for not having their parents. So, at that very young age, I assumed the role of their parent: I felt responsible for them, I helped mom in the kitchen, never fell asleep until both parents were safely home (both were working very long hours), I made sure I kept my word so they would not have to worry about me, and when my sister was born I assumed the role of the third parent. I never thought of my behavior being unusual, as we did not have too many people coming to our house or whose homes we visited. At the time, everybody was working very long hours in Romania building up a country destroyed by World War II.

The next image I see is one of me, at my first kindergarten in Bucharest, desperately crying in a big room full of small beds. I could not communicate with anyone as I spoke only Hungarian and everybody in Bucharest spoke only Romanian. They did not know what to do with me as I was too disruptive, so I was isolated alone in the bedroom. In Transylvania I had my mom and my aunt fussing over me. In Bucharest I had to be put right away into a kindergarten, six days a week, as both my parents were working, and there was no loving aunt to take care of me.

The next scene I see is of me returning from the summer camp with the same kindergarten. I had friends by then. Somehow I succeeded to communicate with them in a very strange self-made language, a combination of Hungarian words with

Romanian suffixes and Romanian words with Hungarian suffixes. When I arrived home, I was concerned of speaking with my parents as they always encouraged me to speak correctly. I was completely quiet on the way home, just making 'yes' and 'no' head movements. At home, in a moment of forgetfulness, I finally said a few words and my parents hugged me crying and repeating: 'We thought you went mute from the shock of being in the camp, but you didn't!' After that, they changed the kindergarten to one with fewer children and a much kinder director, who helped me learn the Romanian language very fast. I have fond memories of all the staff at the second kindergarten, the activities we had when we were in the city, and especially the magical summers when we went into the mountains, to avoid the hot Bucharest summers. It was at that kindergarten, at age five, where I met my best childhood friend and future husband.

I can see a whole film of the lazy summer days, running after butterflies, getting sweets from the kitchen because I was speaking Hungarian [the whole kitchen staff was Hungarian], and learning interesting things about the trees and plants, and how to use the plants to make different handcrafts.

From all those summers one stands out: the one when I was told that I will have the sibling I so much wanted. I even had HER name picked out, and when my parents asked what name to give the baby if it is a boy, I replied with the certainty only a child can have: 'It will be a girl!' and I continued playing. My parents were lucky (me too!), it was indeed a girl. I wonder what would have happened if it had been a boy?!

The next scenes are with me helping to take care of my sister, showing her off to my friends, and taking her everywhere I could. My parents were very smart: they played up the fact that I was a 'big sister', so I was extremely proud of that role and played it to the hilt. I even started cooking at age seven because my sister would eat with gusto anything I cooked. She was a picky eater otherwise.

A lot of images of me feeding my sister are passing by. It was quite an assignment to feed her. Now, years later, I understand that she could not eat because she took so many antibiotics due to constant ear, throat, and sinus infections."

"Interesting. It sounds like you really liked being the big sister, but we will talk about that later. Can you just try to see what happened to YOU? How was the relationship with your parents? Look at the times you spent with them."

"Sorry, I feel that my sister was such a big part of my youth. She defined it... Okay, I am going back to my memories with my parents. I can see two of them dancing together every New Year's Eve. My dad was always doing everything he could to make mom happy. Half a century later I would realize that my mom had severe PTSD[7] because of what she went through during the war[8], but at the time no one even knew that PTSD existed.

My parents decided to have another child so I would not be alone. Unfortunately, my sister's arrival proved to be emotionally overwhelming for my mother and she would easily get very upset. As she worked full time, we were taken care of by young girls – 15 to 18 years old – who came from Transylvania. In those times it was a rite of passage

---

[7] PTSD [Post-Traumatic Stress Disorder] is a mental disorder that can develop after a person is exposed to a traumatic event, such as sexual assault, warfare, traffic collisions, or other threats on a person's life. Symptoms may include disturbing thoughts, feelings, or dreams related to the events, mental or physical distress to trauma-related cues, attempts to avoid trauma-related cues, alterations in how a person thinks and feels, and an increase in the fight-or-flight response. [Wikipedia.org]

[8] The night before my father and mother had to go into the Budapest ghetto [the gathering place before deportation to extermination or work camps] a Christian schoolmate of my father offered my mom his sister's documents. He told them: "My sister just passed away. We are going to bury her in secret for now. With these documents Eve [my mom] does not have to go to the ghetto." The Good Samaritan even offered his apartment to my mom to hide in and sent her a letter from the front with "Dear Sister", which later would save my mother's life. As the apartment was in an industrial area of Budapest, my mother could not move during the day for fear of being detected and both she and her benefactor being executed. It did not help that the area was bombarded every day....

for these young girls to learn from a family in a big city how to manage their future families. They would learn how to cook, take care of the house, and most importantly how to take care of a baby. Once they gained the necessary knowledge, these girls were ready to get married and have their own families, with the city experience being an asset.

Unfortunately, because these girls were young, they could be highly irresponsible at times. In 1952 Romania was still fighting food shortages. The girls would invite young fellows to our place and feed them with the food that was intended for us. My mom would shop at the farmers' market early in the morning, before going to work. By the time she got home from work, she would find the food had disappeared and the girls claimed I ate it all. As my mom was afraid to say anything to the girls for fear that they would leave, I was the only available outlet for her anger. She used to take my long braids, twist them around her arm then bang my head into the stucco wall or a cabinet. Once her anger discharged, my mom would leave me, deeply confused, only to return a while later and tell me how much she loved me. [I fully believe that she indeed loved me and that she could not contain her anger due to PTSD.] Thus began the unhealthy pattern of connecting love and abuse.

Later, after I got married, this pattern would play out again and again both in my family and professional life.

Sometimes my mom would ask my father to discipline me, because my father was adamant about not hitting my head. So my father would take me to another room and ask me to shout as if he were beating me, but I could not lie [one of my GREAT shortcomings], so I would ask my dad to just go ahead and proceed with the necessary beating to my behind, so my mom could calm down knowing that I was disciplined.

My dad was much less impacted by the Holocaust. He was born in a German city in Transylvania, so he spoke German very well. Also, as it was his habit all his life, he took with him to the forced labor camp a set of tools so he would be able to do repairs. Both the language and the tools came in handy when, in the camp, the guards asked who could do repairs. He ended up doing repairs, not only for the camp, but also for the guards' families, which meant from time to time an additional piece of bread or a bowl of soup, the difference between life and death by starvation. Another help for easier weathering the deportation was the fact that my father was with a friend, hence he was not stuck facing the terrible times[9] alone.

My dad had few anger outbursts and in his case I usually knew what generated it, so it was not so bad. Twice I ended up with my behind so red from being disciplined that I could not sit down in school. I would hold on to the desk to keep myself from touching the seat. I remember one time it was a misunderstanding connected with my first grade teacher's explanation of the homework, which resulted in me repeatedly messing up the way I was drawing the letters 'l' and 'e', which were presented to us as the 'big smoke' and 'small smoke', so that is what I was drawing. I was at home alone at the time and my father came home several times from the office to check on me, every time finding me doing the same thing, until he could not take it anymore and let me go to school with the homework done the way I understood it. Another time, in the fifth grade, I was obsessive about some book of math problems I needed to prepare for a math competition. My father was trying to have dinner, while I continued to insist that I needed the money right away. He did not ask why, and I missed telling him that there were only a few copies of the book and if I did not pick them up by a certain time, they would be sold. After being 'disciplined', my father expressed his frustration of

---

[9] After the war, my father's friend from the camp became the first Hungarian ambassador to the USA.

not being able to have a peaceful dinner. I finally told him the book was probably sold because it was on hold only until a certain time. Luckily, once I got the money from my father I was still able to buy the book. The store manager knew me as an avid reader, and they held the book a bit longer.

The worst beating I got when I was twenty-two. I did not know at the time, but my father had to make a list of people to be laid off. At that time in Romania, a person laid off was practically left jobless as there was no way of finding out about job openings or to move freely from one city to another. My father, being very kind by nature, worked very hard to find placements for all the people he had to put on the list, so by the end of the exercise he was exhausted. It was a minor event that sparked his anger, but all the accumulated pain came out and I ended up being beaten so badly I woke up in the hospital, missing the rest of the university studies for that year. The biggest impact though was not the beating, but my terrible fear that my dad could 'wake up' and realize what he was doing. I was the only one in the family who knew that he had heart problems and was in danger of having a heart attack at any time. As he needed to have somebody give him nitroglycerin in case of a heart attack, he decided that I was the best to help him out. As such, once I realized that my dad was practically in an altered state I just went into a fetal position covering my head and stayed quiet, so my father would not get the shock of realizing what he was doing. Eventually I blacked out and I came to in the hospital where I stayed for a while. I could not read, as I had double vision with two perfect images shifted horizontally about 1 in (2.5 cm) apart. I also had terrible headaches and even when I read, I could not make sense of anything. My father came to the hospital and explained to me repeatedly why he was so angry and asked for forgiveness, but I would just listen to him, not understanding anything, then falling back to sleep. I nearly stopped my engineering studies, but my aunt's loving care[10], the unconditional help from my father[11], and the care of a knowledgeable eye doctor, put my life back on track.

I was never upset with my dad, as I understood why it all happened."

Like in a dream I heard Isabelle: "As you are talking, I keep hearing about your dad a lot, but not as much

---

[10] I lived with my aunt and her family for a couple of month, until I was able to understand things again. Many years later, I understood that what she did was the only way to extinguish the "trauma response" that could have caused PTSD in the long run. To this day I do not know if it was her experience as a doctor or her unconditional love for me that made her do it.

[11] My father repeatedly read and explained the exam material for me, so I would be able to pass at least some of my exams in the summer session.

about your mother. Why is that?! Can you figure it out?"

"My relationship with my dad was not only one from father to child, but also one of mentor to mentee. He was the reason I became an engineer. He was very busy working two jobs while I was young, but his time with us, his daughters, was always fun. I could learn new things from him or be part of a kind prank played on me or my sister.

My mom worked a lot and was always so tired that she would fall asleep as soon as she sat down. She was always overstressed, trying to manage work and family, despite my father's help.

For some reason, my mom did not like the fact that I had a strong character. I was a good kid (as she would later tell me): responsible, reliable, good student, and caring sibling, but somehow she was very tough on me. She always misinterpreted my behavior in a negative way, as if trying to find fault with everything I was doing. If I was sick, she would accuse me of faking it, like when I had a traumatic brain injury that made me incapable to function and she told all our relatives that I was perfectly well, just making it up. This latter story would make my loving aunt call me repeatedly long distance and give me speeches on the topic of 'getting hold of myself', which I obviously could not. Another time, when my in-laws sent us some gifts through my parents and they were lost, I was accused again of having forgotten that I received them, which caused a lot of problems in my marriage and the anger of my relatives. In that case, the only person who acted in a reasonable fashion was my father's sister who believed me. I was always on my mother's bad side. Any time something went wrong, I was unjustly accused of being the source of the problem."

"As you are looking back at your childhood do you remember anything positive about it? Look through your memories." I heard Isabelle telling me.

"Oh yes! There were many positive things." I replied, then continued: "I always knew that my parents loved us, and they did their best to take care of us. I understood from a very young age that it was very hard for them as they did not have any help from grandparents or siblings[12]. They used to say that if they could have somebody reliable to just come by from time to time to check on us, it would make a world of difference. But they did not have anyone"

"Look back at your life. How did your relationship with your parents impact your life?" I heard Isabelle asking me again.

---

[12] We lived in a different city from where all our relatives lived, and all my grandparents were dead.

"I believe I was lucky to have loving parents. I was relatively safe. I knew that either of them would protect me against anything bad from the outside world. At the same time, the fact that I assumed the role of parent to my parents made me responsible from a very young age. While other kids must be cajoled to do their homework, for me it was a way to bring my parents happiness, and that was worth any effort.

My mother's PTSD outbursts were very painful both physically and emotionally. It also made me believe that maybe I was not my mother's child, but a child brought by my father into the family. This was due to both resembling my father's side of the family, and the fact that he treated me with the unconditional love of a true father. I felt protected by him. Mom always praised my dad (as dad did mom), so I ended up always watching what dad was doing and wanting to do the same things. I eventually ended up being a home repair wizard by age 12, when my dad ceded to me his position as the family repair man. This handiness with tools, eventually made me go into engineering, which made my father proud.

My mother was very proud of me too. She liked dressing me up, and showing me off, which in fact was an additional source of confusion when she would berate me in private.

Before my mom passed away I asked her if I was a bad kid. She told me: 'To the contrary. You were very responsible. I could always count on your promises. If you promised to do something it was usually done perfectly and ahead of time.' In our very last discussion, she asked me for forgiveness. I told her I knew she did the best she could, and I always believed that.

In the end, the heritage from my parents is one of unconditional love, respect for others, a deep sense of responsibility, and a constant striving to improve myself.

My mother also taught me a lot about how to take care of my son and, once she was no longer pressed by the demands of a job and became a 'visiting grandmother', her advice was right to the point and always helpful.

My father taught me to love people and always help as much as I could. He inspired me to go into engineering and was proud of my achievements."

"So, if you would have to define the role of your parents in your development as an individual, how would you rate them?" I heard Isabelle's voice in the distance.

"I am deeply grateful to them for providing a strong moral compass, teaching me good work ethics and how to fight to achieve my life goals, for giving me their wisdom, and especially for going past their level of comfort and deciding to give me a sister, in spite of all the additional work and expense[13] involved in that decision."

"Take a minute to revisit your memories. Is there anything else you need to bring up today related to your parents, anything that needs to be clarified?"

"No, I think I understand now everything related to my parents. I am ready to come back."

"So, step through the mirror again and find yourself in the gazebo. Look again at the beautiful trees and start walking the path back, being more and more aware of your physical body…. When you are ready, just gently open your eyes and come back into the room."

As soon as I opened my eyes, I heard Isabelle's voice: "Congratulations! You did a wonderful job. See you next time for another interesting journey."

A bit dazed and my heart full of gratitude for my parents, I left Isabelle's office. It was winter outside,

---

[13] Despite my father working two jobs, and my mom working full time, my parents always had to be very careful with money. In those times, the salaries, even for professionals, were low, there were constant food shortages, and while medical care was officially free, you had to pay doctors under the table, or you would not get appointments when you needed them.

so night was falling, but my heart was still full of the image of that beautiful garden filled with leafy trees and colorful flowers.

Gaining Insight into One's Childhood

Work through this questionnaire for each person who was like a parent for you. For example, if you were raised by an aunt or uncle, they would be your "parents". If you were in foster care, do the exercise for each family you were a part of.

My father/mother………… was……………………………..

…………………………………………………………………………..

…………………………………………………………………………..

[Fill in the name and general description, such as: "My father, Oswald, who I lived with from age 5 to 11, was a kind, considerate, loving man."]

The negative memories I have about……………… are:

1. ……………………………………………………………
   ……………………………………………………………
   ……………………………………………………………
2. ……………………………………………………………
   ……………………………………………………………
   ……………………………………………………………
3. ……………………………………………………………
   ……………………………………………………………
   ……………………………………………………………
4. ……………………………………………………………
   ……………………………………………………………

5. ....

Because of the negative experiences I had with………
I decided:

1. ....

2. ....

3. ....

4. ....

5. ....

[For example: because of my father's abusive behavior, I decided I was worthless, which impacted later my relationships.]

My positive life decisions as a result of my negative experiences connected with…………………………are:

1. ....
....
....

2. ....
....
....

3. ....
....
....

4. ....
....
....

5. ....
....
....

[For example: because of the negative experience of being physically disciplined by my father, I decided never to do that to my children; because of the confusion generated by the seemingly random physical punishment I decided I will always make sure my children understand why they were disciplined...]

The positive memories related to ……………. are:

1. ....
....
....

2. ....
....

3. ....
....
....

4. ....
....
....

5. ....
....
....

Because of the positive experiences I had with..........
I decided:

1. ....
....
....

2. ....
....
....

3. ....
....
....

4. ....
....
....

5. ....
....
....

[For example: because of my positive experience with my father who was kind, helpful, and had a can-do attitude whenever he had to do something, I decided I will do the same.]

The top five blessings that come from my experiences with ……………. are:

1. …………………………………………………………………
   …………………………………………………………………
   …………………………………………………………………
2. …………………………………………………………………
   …………………………………………………………………
   …………………………………………………………………
3. …………………………………………………………………
   …………………………………………………………………
   …………………………………………………………………
4. …………………………………………………………………
   …………………………………………………………………
   …………………………………………………………………
5. …………………………………………………………………
   …………………………………………………………………
   …………………………………………………………………

[For example: I learned to be kind to others, I learned to have a can-do attitude, and I learned to be supportive.]

It is most important to understand that even the negative events in our lives can have a positive impact. It all depends whether we choose to look at our life experiences as teachable moments, or if we prefer to drown in self-pity[14].

---

[14] The most extreme examples of using negative life experiences in a positive way are those of people severely abused, such as in the case of Dave Pelzer, the author of "A Child Called 'It'".

Being a Sister

ભ્જી

"Are you ready to talk about being a sister?" asked Isabelle as soon as she saw me.

"Yes, I look forward to it. Our relationship was both a rewarding and, at the same time, a painful one. I truly hope to figure it out."

"What do you mean?" asked Isabelle inviting me into her office.

"I always considered my sister as a gift. When she was little, I took care of her as if she was my own child. Once we grew up, we became friends, even taking her on vacations with my family.

Something happened though once I left the country. Our history was completely changed in her mind and she always tried to convince me that I hated her for displacing me in our parents' attention, when she was born. I have no idea where this came from[15]. It was extremely painful every time we had that

---

[15] It might have originated with my mother. Because of her Holocaust experience, my mother had a deep fear of losing us. As such, she became possessive of us, even more of my sister after I left. Her relationship with my sister ended up being a symbiotic one, as she took total control of my sister's life.

discussion. In addition, she seemed to have erased all the positive memories from our childhood, as if only bad things happened. It was as if she wanted to justify something."

"Is your sister still alive?" asked Isabelle next.

"No. She passed away due to cancer. Her final act was that, despite me being her main caretaker during her battle with cancer, she gifted all her estate to others."

"Wow! That must have really hit you in the gut. You really need some closure on this! Let us start."

With that, Isabelle settled in her chair, inviting me to do the same. Soon enough, under her guidance, I was back in the enchanted garden, climbing the steps of the gazebo.

"Do you see the mirror marked 'Being a Sister'?"

"Yes", I replied. "I am just about to step through."

"Go ahead. This is YOUR life. ... and as you step inside the mirror, see the movie of your significant memories related to your sister."

I followed Isabelle's directions and I started replaying the memories: the joy of having a sister, the worry when she repeatedly got sick when she was only four months old, me constantly begging my parents to let me take care of her during the night. My parents were very tired from the sleepless nights, but they would not let me take over Grace's care. I was only seven. Finally, one time when my sister was better, my parents left her in my care. I listened to her breathing and the first time she made a sound, I took her out of her crib, changed her diapers, and took her into my bed. I left most of the space for my sister to make sure I did not by mistake roll over her, and we went to sleep peacefully until the following morning.

My parents told me the rest of the story when I grew up. They woke surprised that Grace did not cry during the night and they could have a restful sleep. But when my mom came into my room the next morning, she got the scare of her life: there was no baby in the crib! Looking around, after the first shock, she noticed both of us sleeping peacefully in my bed. I was never again allowed to oversee my sister during the night. My parents were afraid of me rolling over her.

Next I see myself cooking for my sister. She was a picky eater, but she ate everything I cooked for her. I asked my parents to teach me to cook but, as a seven-year-old, they did not want me working with the gas stove. So, after watching carefully how the adults cooked, I repeated the steps. The problem was that I tried to make polenta, but I was given only the chaff left after passing the corn meal through the sieve. Luckily mom noticed in time that I was just about to feed my sister my version of polenta.[16]

Next I see myself going to be registered for the first grade. Being born in April I could start school at six and a half or a year later. I begged my parents to let me stay home for one more year so I could play with Grace. As a last resort I promised them, if they let me stay home one more year, I would be a very good student. That finally worked! I happily started school a year later, and I kept my promise.

I also remember sleeping in the same room with my sister and telling her bedtime stories invented by me. I even ended up writing for her a whole notebook full of fairytales. Eventually I destroyed the book the day my parents found it. I considered it a serious invasion of my privacy as the stories were intended only for my sister.

Years passed and my sister started to study violin, so we ended up preparing for finals at the same time. I found myself reading the same paragraph again and again as my sister was repeating the same piece of music again and again. But we made it.

I was considerably older. Six and a half years at that age is significant, so I became the elder among my

---

[16] Polenta is made by boiling corn meal in salted water. It is quite tasty as a side, with cold milk, or with farmer's cheese and sour cream.

cousins, being a reliable babysitter when I would visit my aunt in summer. She had two children just a bit younger than my sister, so I would take them and Grace with me everywhere I could. I loved them and enjoyed watching them play together.

My sister and my aunt's daughter became lifelong friends. I found out only many years later, when I was in my sixties, that I was considered intimidating, not only by my sister and my aunt's children, but also by my uncle's children, who were even younger.

Next I can see boys coming to visit me and my sister reporting back to mom what she was seeing through the keyhole. It wasn't much to see, but I was 'under control'. This worked also in my favor. Our parents used to discuss important decisions in the mornings while getting ready for work. Grace was always ready and listening through the keyhole, and reported back to me.

While we had the usual fights between siblings, we were close. When it came to my wedding it was a tug of war between my mother and my future mother-in-law. My mom did not want me to marry my future husband and as such she wanted no part in preparing me for my wedding. When she invited our relatives, who all still lived in Transylvania, she gave them the date of the wedding with the caveat that the wedding will be on the given date, unless they can convince me not to marry. The result was none of my cousins came to the wedding. I would have loved to have them with me on my Big Day.

As for my wedding dress and shoes, it was my sister who came with me to buy them. It was interesting that my mom had no problem going with my sister and buying her a dress and shoes for the wedding.

I was very grateful to my sister, as I considered it painful not to have my mother share my life-changing day. My sister's support softened the blow. My dad was not good at buying women's clothes, but he was staunchly on my side. The only thing he said half-jokingly at the city hall[17] was 'There is the door. You can still run away if you change your mind.' I did not run away...

The next scene I can see is me looking at my newborn son and being surprised that my feelings toward him were very much like the ones I had for my sister. I knew immediately how to take care of him as I had practiced extensively on my sister.

Grace loved my son. As in Romania it was considered bad luck to buy baby clothes before the baby was born[18] we had to go and buy my son stuff as soon as I got home from the hospital. To my sister's delight,

---

[17] In Romania at the time, the city hall weddings were the only ones recognized.

[18] Probably originated in the fact that the child mortality in those days was high.

we left my son in her care. As we were shopping, I suddenly had a strong feeling that we had to return home as something demanded our attention. When Grace opened the door, we did not know what to do, laugh or cry. There was my sister crying while holding our son whose diapers were open, freely flowing off him. Upon enquiring what was going on, Grace told us she wanted to hold the baby as soon as we left, so she gently picked up our son who was fast asleep. He started to cry, so my sister assumed he needed a diaper change, but under pressure, she forgot how to do it, hence the flowing diapers. Once we found out that nothing tragic was happening, we all had a good laugh and my sister promised not to pick Johnny up next time she was in charge and he was asleep.

The next memory is going on vacation with my husband, my son, and my sister, to the Black Sea shore. She was the second child for us, and I was happy my husband accepted her as such.

Soon after returning from vacation my sister had an accident that nearly ended her young life. A drunk driver got onto the sidewalk where my sister was happily chatting with her friends after a school dance. Three students were hit that evening. One of them died on the spot, after being literally imprinted on the wall of the building that stopped the car. My sister had several broken ribs, a smashed right femur, and a broken pelvis. She was taken to the hospital emergency room by some strangers who saw the accident happening. The third youngster was so shocked, he wandered the city streets until early morning and, when he got home, he could not tell his parents what exactly happened.

When I saw Grace in the hospital for the first time I was terrified I would lose her but, with mom's help, she fought her way back. While in the hospital, mom was with Grace day and night, hardly sleeping for months and, once home, mom became Grace's full time caretaker. My part in this was to keep my parents' morale up, by frequently visiting with my toddler.

I still have a sweet picture of my sister and my son learning to walk at the same time. Yes, my sister needed to relearn to walk, after going through multiple surgeries to repair her broken leg that also got infected.

I do not know when the break in our relationship happened. My husband defected from Romania in 1974 and my son and I immigrated to Israel in 1977. It was not easy to leave Romania in those days, so my husband decided to defect when he got a scholarship in England. I knew at the time he left that he was not planning on coming back. We thought we would be apart for a maximum of six months, but it ended up being two and a half years.

The only other person in the family who knew my husband's plan to defect was my dad. Just before my husband's defection my father had a very serious surgery, so we had to go to the hospital to tell him our plans. My dad wished Peter good luck and promised him to protect me as much as he could. He kept his promise at a great price. It was the first time in many years of marriage that my father was not completely open with my mother and mom never forgave him for that. She was afraid of the consequences of my husband's defection would have on my sister, but luckily she was not affected.

I do not know if that was the start of the break in my relationship with my sister, or when she first visited us in Canada. Finding that I could not get employment in my profession[19] (computer engineering) in Israel, we applied for immigration to Canada and Australia. We got accepted by both and decided to immigrate once more, this time to Canada.

Once in Canada, from the first money we could save, we sent a ticket so my sister could visit us, after her summer course in France. I missed my sister badly, as she was an integral part of my young family before

---

[19] I was considered a security risk because my parents and sister were still in Romania.

immigration. We literally spent all our savings in order to bring her to visit us.

First thing she told us when she came into our home was how cheap our furniture and drapes looked. I was deeply hurt as we saved every penny we could so we could buy her ticket. We took her around and had a good time. At the end, before Grace left, we took my her to the most expensive jewelry store in Toronto and asked her to choose a ring as a gift to take home. (It would take many years before we bought any jewelry for me.) She would give away the ring as soon as she got home, after somebody told her it was bad luck because the ring she chose had a pearl in it.

A few days before leaving Toronto, out of the blue, my sister declared that she had no intention of returning to Romania. When we told her that we were still struggling, not on our feet yet, so it would be a much better idea to go back, find a nice guy and emigrate with him as the ideas about marriage in the west were not exactly what she was used to, my sister dropped another bomb: she told us that the school year had already started so she had no job to go back to.

Luckily, with the help of my in-laws, we were able to get my sister's job back and she was not punished for her transgression of staying abroad past the start of the school year. After that my sister always brought up the fact that we were heartless to send her back to Romania.

Some years later my parents visited us. By that time, we lived in a townhouse and we had a Buick in our driveway. Once my mom saw that, she decided that we were stinking rich, as in Romania owning both a house and a Buick were possible only for the very well to do people. I tried to explain to her that in fact both of those were owned mostly by the bank, but because in those times in Romania one bought things with all the money down, she did not understand the concept. Every time we went out to the mall she wanted to buy every expensive item in sight, and because I kept telling her we could not afford it, she would become very upset. Knowing that I was generous by nature, she decided that my husband was at fault, so the relationship between the two of them became very strained, despite my father's efforts to moderate.

I believe that, when my mom returned to Romania upset because how cheap we were, she might have influenced my sister's views, who readily embraced mom's take on things, being already angry about having to return to Romania when she visited us.

Eventually Grace got married and followed her husband to the United States. The first year she was in the U.S., my parents visited us again. At the same time, because my extensive work with the research branch of our company headquartered in Minnesota, I was asked to relocate to the States. The relocation was planned for the same time my parents were scheduled to visit. Because it was very difficult to obtain a visa to travel outside Romania, we decided not to postpone my parents' visit. We made the move to the U.S. with my parents in tow, my company being very generous with the moving expenses as they needed me in the U.S. as soon as possible. The demand for my work with the budding very large-scale integrated (VLSI) technology[20] definition was much too great.

Unfortunately, the employment promised for my husband, as a condition for me accepting to move, did not work out as originally planned and my husband had to start looking for a job.

So my parents would not feel they were a burden, Peter told them we could survive even if he did not work for a long time[21] which, for my mom, again sounded like: 'they are stinking rich', and it ended up

---

[20] This was the technology that later enabled the notebook, iPhone, and iPad designs.

[21] In fact, we had serious financial problems. I even entertained the idea of finding a second job, despite the long hours I was already spending at the office. As my husband could not find a job, we were in danger of losing our home. Luckily, my boss found out about it and he obtained for me a salary increase that saved us. I am forever grateful for his kindness!

the same pattern of wanting to buy everything expensive and blaming my husband for not doing so.

Everything came to a head just before Christmas that year. My parents were visiting since July and my mom, sick and tired of our cheapness, wanted to go and visit my sister. We offered to buy her a ticket, but she demanded that we buy one for my father too, which we could not afford at the time. I tried to explain to my mom that my sister and her new husband needed time together as a couple, that my sister just started work and they needed to settle, and that the one-bedroom apartment my sister had at the time was too small for all of them, while they had a comfortable in-law apartment in our home specially bought for their comfort, but nothing helped. I suggested an alternative: we could have my sister and her husband over for the holidays and we could spend time together. I would cook and we would all have a good time.

My mom had other plans, and she was quite creative. As soon as my sister arrived, my mom and my sister went and bought some food and drinks despite having in the house everything they liked to eat, then settled in the lower level in-law apartment talking. Every time I went there they stopped talking and looked at me as if I was an intruder. At some point, I noticed a lot of commotion and when I went to enquire what was going on and tell them the dinner was ready, I was told that my parents, my sister, and her husband were leaving because my husband hurt my dad's feeling. They packed in a hurry and they were out the door in no time, leaving me perplexed. To complete her work, my mother cursed me and my family on her way out. After they left my son, my husband, and I literally huddled together holding on to each other for dear life because the energy in the house was very heavy.

After that, my relationship with my birth family was totally changed. My parents eventually decided to leave Romania by asking for a tourist visa and never returning from the trip. They left behind everything they worked for all their lives. The only things we eventually saved were some technical books my father cherished that I collected when I later visited Romania.

My parents lived with my sister who, in time, bought a nice home. I visited them every time I could, but the relationship with my husband was pretty much broken. Every time I went there I would be in tears. While my father was delighted to see me, my mom and my sister treated me like the 'scum of the earth', bringing me to tears. When my father was diagnosed with cancer, my mom did everything not to let me help him in any way, treating me with a jealousy fit for a mistress, not her own child. (This raised further questions in my mind regarding whether she was my birth mother.) My sister pretty much followed my mother's lead, so I promised myself, when my father died, that I will never talk to them again... but I did, justifying it with the fact that I had only one mother and one sister and I did not want to lose them.

I tried to help them every way I could, from having mom over so my sister could have time off, to taking my vacations when my sister traveled. Interestingly, once my dad passed away, my mother and sister started treating me somewhat better, but still my sister found a special pleasure in finding fault in everything connected with me: from the way I was choosing to manage my money, to my classic taste in dresses. As I had difficulty finding elegant clothing for my body type, I started sewing my own dresses. People thought I was buying my dresses in boutiques, but Grace always criticized me.

Grace's biggest wish, even after my parents passed away, was to see me divorced and hated the fact that I considered my husband's and my son's care a priority. The holiday season arrived not long after my mother passed away. I suggested that Grace come and spend time with us, but she insisted I leave my son and husband and spend the holidays with her. As I refused, she checked herself into the hospital, so I would feel guilty, and had all sorts of tests done while the doctors could not find anything wrong with her.

After a few years, when my sister was diagnosed with cancer I became her main physical support. Still, she was angry at me. She did not look at what I was doing, instead always looking for the stuff she wanted me to do but I could not provide. She wanted me to be with her when she had her chemo sessions and would not hear about the fact that, even at a distance, as a healer, I was absorbing the toxicity of the treatments and I felt quite sick from it. Every time she had a chemo session I worked protecting her vital organs[22], a fact that was later independently confirmed by a healer she knew. Still my sister brought up repeatedly the fact that I did not hold her hand when she had chemo.

Her cancer went in remission for four years, only to appear again in a more virulent form[23].

---

[22] Usually chemotherapy causes damage to the vital organs. After finishing chemo, my sister's healer friend was very surprised to find all my sister's organs in perfect health. Because of the healing work of protecting my sister's organs I was nauseous, had headaches, and felt tired, all through the time my sister was going through her chemotherapy. I had painful gallbladder attacks every time I tried to eat the smallest amount of fatty food. Interestingly, three days after her passing, the green coating on my tongue (a sign of liver distress) disappeared and I was able to eat fried food with no discomfort. Gaining back my usual energy level took quite some more time.

[23] This is not unusual as every chemotherapy has as a side effect cancer. Also, chemo destroys the immune system. It is basically a race between which cells die first from toxicity: the cancerous cells or the good ones.

During the second bout with cancer my sister was subjected to experimental treatments that many times left her so weak she could hardly function, but her sense of duty kicked in and she continued working until shortly before her death.

While during my sister's first bout with cancer I was still married, during the second one, my life was basically on hold and I traveled to be with my sister whenever she needed it, even when I was still recovering from a serious surgery and walking with a cane. But that was not enough, again and again being told the list of my wrongdoings. I was getting lectures on every aspect of my life: from not being a good parent, to being married too long, to why I had the home I had. Everything I did was wrong, including the fact that I had a positive outlook on life. It seemed everything I said or did was an opportunity to find fault with me. It was painful, but I stayed by Grace as she had no one else to help her. I knew the day she would stop teaching (she was an amazingly talented teacher) her life would be over. As she was divorced and had no children of her own, I was the only person who could be there for her.

She was also extremely competitive with me. If I bought something, she had to buy something bigger/more expensive. I begged her to stop spending so much as I had a strong feeling her income could not support her habits, but she would not listen. One way to allay her guilt of spending was to ask me to buy her something then buying something 'to return the favor'. Once I understood the game I started refusing to accept any' gifts' from her and tried not to tell her about things that I bought.

While in the hospital for her last round of treatments, Grace decided to make up a will that could have caused serious friction between me and my son. I was deeply hurt, but I decided to continue taking care of her. I realized it was her competitiveness that made her do it.

At the end, I think Grace might have had an inkling of what she did. She noticed that everybody she considered as her favorites had gone on vacation and only I was left by her side. Seeing her fear of death, I carefully eased myself into Grace's bed and hugged her the way I used to when she was a child. The last words she was able to say were 'Thank you, sis!'[24] When she passed a few days later, I was at peace that my sister had the best care I could provide, and I was indeed a true sister to the end."

---

[24] By the end, the cancer had spread in my sister's spine and brain. This helped her not to feel pain, which was a blessing, but also took away her capability to speak and control her bodily functions.

"Now that you looked in depth at your relationship with your sister, are you sorry you wanted to have a sister?" I heard Isabelle's question like in a dream.

"Not for a moment. I admired Grace for her achievements, for her valiant fight to recover after her terrible accident when she was young, and for her fight to stay on her feet despite her cancer. I admired her talent to relate to people as if each one was the most important person in the world, and for her talent as a teacher. I was also grateful for helping our parents. I wish she would have been more open to accept what I had learned from my practice helping people with cancer, but I had to learn to be at peace with her life choices.

Always dreaming to live the life of a rich person, my sister convinced herself that money would come into her life whenever she needed it, so she never considered seriously saving for retirement, or properly managing her money. She also compared herself with me and, as such, could not truly appreciate her own accomplishments as a teacher who changed many lives for the better. She considered herself 'not too smart' because she was not good at math. As much as I explained to her that it was the equivalent of me being miserable because I could not play the violin or even hold a tune, it did not make any difference. I miss her every day, as she was more like my child than my sister, but there is nothing I can do about it."

"What did you learn from your sister?" I heard Isabelle asking.

"I learned to accept with gratitude whatever people are doing for me and giving without expecting anything in return. I learned that people have their own lives and I must respect their decisions, even if that is painful for me. My sister's life experience reinforced what I learned from so many others: negative emotions are more damaging than a bad diet, lack of sleep, or any other negative habit. Above all, I had a lesson in forgiveness as I had a choice to be angry at my sister for the way she treated me or working on letting go of the pain she caused and continuing to do what my conscience was directing me to do. I am grateful I chose the path of forgiveness as it allowed me to give my sister the loving care she needed and, even after her passing, I was able to take care of her estate as if it was mine to inherit."

"Is there anything else you need to deal with related to your sister?" Isabelle asked again.

"While the pain of losing her still lingers, I think I am done for now. I would like though to meet her in the garden on my way back, if you don't mind."

"No problem! It is your session, so if you want to talk with your sister, you can do it."

"I am in the gazebo. Now I am walking back. I find myself in the Bronx Botanical Garden where we walked together the last spring she was alive. I can see my sister! I feel so happy!!! She is fine. She is talking to me; I must get closer to understand. She is walking toward me too! She tells me she is well, she has no more pain, and she can talk again. She is with our parents and she feels safe and happy to have left all the chemo toxicity behind. She is reading again and looks forward to reading my next book. Now she understands things better. She knows a lot of truths I was telling her about. She knows I wanted her best.... We are hugging... She must go now.... She is grateful for the meeting... so am I. We hug for a while, then she walks away smiling.... I am ready to come back now."

"Wow, what a session! This was some important stuff you went through. How nice to have met your sister at the end. Do you feel the need to share anything else?" asked Isabelle as I opened my eyes.

"No. Not really. I feel the need to be quiet and absorb the session. Thank you so much for your help. I look forward to our next session."

"Me too!" replied Isabelle as she walked me to the door.

Gaining Insight into Being a Sibling

Work through this questionnaire for each person who was like a sister or brother for you. For example, if you were raised by an aunt or uncle, your cousins would have been like your siblings, or if you were an only child, you probably had a very close friend who was like a sibling for you.

My .... was................................

....

....

[For example: "My cousin Andrew was like a brother for me. We did everything together."]

The negative memories I have about.................. are:

1. ....
....
....

2. ....
....
....

3. ....
....
....

4. ....
....

....

5. ....

....

....

Because of the negative experiences I had with………
I decided:

1. ....

....

....

2. ....

....

....

3. ....

....

....

4. ....

....

....

5. ....

....

....

[For example: because I was not invited to Andrew's wedding, I decided never to speak to him again.]

My positive life decisions as a result of my negative experiences connected with…………………………are:

1. ....

2. ....
3. ....
4. ....
5. ....

[For example: when, after 20 years, I finally decided to find out why I was not invited to the wedding, I found out that Andrew also wondered why I did not attend his wedding. (The mistake was with the person who wrote the invitations.) I decided, because of this experience, in similar cases, to always enquire what was going on, so I would avoid miscommunication.

The positive memories related to ……………. are:

1. ....
2. ....

3. ....

4. ....

5. ....

Because of the positive experiences I had with.........
I decided:

1. ....

2. ....

3. ....

4. ....

5. ....

[For example: because of my positive experience with my friend, I decided to use this experience as a lesson for my children, so they would not make the same mistake.]

The top five blessings that come from my experiences with ……………. are:

1. ………………………………………………………………
   ………………………………………………………………
   ………………………………………………………………

2. ………………………………………………………………
   ………………………………………………………………
   ………………………………………………………………

3. ………………………………………………………………
   ………………………………………………………………
   ………………………………………………………………

4. ………………………………………………………………
   ………………………………………………………………
   ………………………………………………………………

5. ………………………………………………………………
   ………………………………………………………………
   ………………………………………………………………

[For example: I had my friend back after many years, I learned not to get upset before I am sure there is reason for it, etc.]

Being a Wife
ಞ

"Hello Cassie! How are you today? cheerfully greeted me Isabelle "Did you think about the information that came through during the past two sessions? Do you believe we need to work some more on those issues?"

"I believe, at least for now, I am done with those aspects of my life and would like us to go on to my life as a wife. It is important for me to figure out where I went wrong. Was there anything I could have done to make things develop differently?"

Isabelle readily agreed. "Then we can proceed to the next 'mirror trip'. I hope you get out of it what you need." With that, she settled in her chair and invited me to do the same.

In no time I was again in my enchanted garden, then climbing the gazebo steps, and finally stepping through the next mirror. Soon I found myself walking with Peter, my kindergarten best friend, on a beautiful winter night after New Year's Eve. We were both well past our kindergarten years. We were in fact nearing the end of our respective university studies. Everything was white and big snowflakes were lazily falling to the ground. It looked like we were walking in one of the beautiful Russian winter fairytales. Our parents were walking ahead of us and we were in a world of our own. Suddenly I had the feeling that we had been friends/partners through many lifetimes, and I found myself dancing with Peter in a 'cosmic dance' among the stars. I do not know how long it lasted and, when it ended, I had a very strong feeling that one day I would marry him.

Next I saw us meeting at the kindergarten when we were barely five. Neither of us had any siblings at the time so we became best friends. I was the older one, by a few months.

We lived very close and, on weekends, we used to go and play at the park together, sometimes just the two of us and other times with my future father-in-law. We never played at Peter's place, as we had to be very quiet not to disturb his mom. It seemed she was either at work or sleeping.

When the weather was bad, we usually played at my home where another friend, Trixie, who was the same age as us, usually joined us. We liked to play 'mom, dad, and child', Peter taking the role of the dad, Trixie was the child, and I was the mom. The dining room table was our 'home' and we spent hours taking care of baby Trixie. I had very strong maternal instincts even then.

Peter and I were the kindergarten favorites as we ate anything they put in front of us, even cod liver oil. (We got a double pickle treat after.) In summer, when the entire kindergarten went into the Transylvanian mountainous area, my best friend was the only one allowed to watch my long hair being washed. It was considered a special treat as my braided hair fell to the middle of my upper legs.

Peter and I were inseparable. When they tried to put me in the girls' room and him in the boys' room to sleep, we cried our eyes out. I ended up sleeping in a smaller boys' room. When it came to bathing, they were bathing one child at each of the two ends of the bathtub, but they had to bathe us together. By the time we were around seven years old, the kindergarten director decided it was time to bathe us separately. We cried again, so we ended up being the last two kids being washed. Once in the bathtub, we tried to figure out why the teachers were so reluctant to bathe us together. When we got too close to the answer we were yanked out of the tub, never to have another bath until we got home.

We were intrigued as to why two good friends could not bathe together. We were good, we ate our food, did not complain about waiting until the end, so why then not bathe together?

Next day we decided to figure it out. When the kids were taken into the woods to learn how to pick the right grass to make baskets and leaves to make purses, we sneaked back to the house and locked ourselves in one of the kids' bathrooms and discussed the important topic of why we could not bathe together. We discussed it for a long time, going step by step through everything that happened the previous night, but in the end we had to give up. We had to accept that we could not find an answer to our question, and no one else was willing to give us an explanation. We promised each other that whoever found out first, would tell the other.

After a couple of years, Peter and his parents moved from the apartment that was close to where I lived, to one that was a long bus ride away from my apartment building. We rarely met after that. When we did, it was at a library, a bookstore, or at a performance, when we would ask each other polite questions about our respective families.

Then, when we were in our third year of university Peter, who was studying economics, needed my father's help to understand some economics concepts. His father tracked down mine and they paid us a visit. I was inclined to leave the apartment as soon as they arrived because, by that time, my parents and their friends tried to fix me up with nice guys, which I hated. My mother shamed me into staying. I was polite, but no sparks.

Then, about a year later, I was crossing the street while solving math problems in my mind and, as such, not watching the traffic. I was crossing at a low visibility point and a driver nearly ran me over. The driver was my old friend Peter.

I have no recollection of the near miss, but years later he told me it was at that point he knew he would marry me. He asked his father to track me down again. We were invited for dinner and ended up having the 'celestial dance' mentioned earlier, when I got the impression I would marry Peter one day.

As it happens, once we finished our studies, we got married and a little more than a year later our son was born.

Unfortunately, right after our wedding, I discovered for the first time the angry version of Peter. He was a totally different person. As he was much taller than I and of a strong built, the outburst scared me. I wondered what I got into by marrying him.

Things went on peacefully until seven months later when he stood up during dinner and pushed me into the wall, holding my hands raised above my head. I was three months pregnant by then. There was absolutely no warning of that coming. It was a sudden switch from a calm discussion to me ending up facing the wall! Once Peter realized what he was doing, he started laughing telling me: 'This is what I used to do to the guys who were taunting me in school.', but I did NOT taunt him.

The scariest part of this experience was that it felt familiar. I was shocked: why such an obviously abusive behavior felt like I was home. It took me years of therapy to finally understand: It was the connection already existing in my psyche between love and abuse due to my mother's habit of wrapping my braids around her arm and then banging my head into the wall, then later telling me how much she loved me.

The abuse from Peter did not stop. Many years later he would justify it by the fact that he was utterly unprepared for marriage. But why did I and Johnny have to pay for it? I always wondered if my mother-in-law was the one who convinced Peter to get married or if it was truly his decision.

In addition to the angry outbursts, during the first and second years of marriage, Peter also had the habit of coming home very late from the office, so I basically took care of the house and our son, in addition to a demanding full time job and my studies for a Ph.D. in computer design engineering.

My days were packed, and I could study only after everyone else went to bed. I passed my exams with flying colors and had my thesis ready. About the same time, Peter's best friend immigrated to Israel and Peter started to pressure me to find a way to leave Romania.

In Romania, even if somebody was married, he needed the parents' official agreement before being allowed to leave the country. If the parents agreed, everyone: the person who wanted to leave and the parents would lose their jobs and became a pariah, no one daring to talk to them. There was no way Peter's parents would consider giving him their blessing! Peter was also an only child and his parents had high positions in the communist government, which made things even more complex. Hence the only way to leave was to defect. Some people left through Yugoslavia by swimming the width of the Danube while being shot at, others crossed the border to Hungary. Peter was lucky. He got a scholarship to go and study marketing in England, and he used the opportunity to defect.

Before Peter left, I became pregnant again. Knowing of his intention to defect, Peter told me that he would not want to leave me behind with two kids, as one was already difficult enough. While Peter never said directly that he did not want a second child, I understood that he was not thrilled about it, so I had an illegal abortion. The emotional impact of the abortion followed me for decades, and only many years of therapy could erase the deep guilt and pain I felt. I was very grateful that I had my son.

Being left behind when Peter defected had many implications for me: my Ph.D. degree which was in its final stage was denied, I was questioned at my workplace, at Peter's workplace, at the city police, and by Securitate - corresponding to the FBI in the U.S. Everybody wanted to find out if I knew about Peter's defection ahead of time, as that was considered treason, and I would have been thrown in jail for several years. To make things even more interesting, when my in-laws were questioned by the police my mother-in-law told them her son would not have left without my approval[25].

Being apart was very difficult, especially since at work I was sidelined, never again being allowed to do design work. I was given technical specifications in German that I had to translate to Romanian. While this was happening, I had several people spying on me, in addition to getting all my letters with parts cut out of them.

---

[25] At the end of my interview with the city police, I asked them to do whatever they want with me but to leave the parents alone as they were old and had heart problems, and as such the police could end up literally killing them. When the policeman heard this, he told me that it was interesting how different my position was versus that of my mother-in-law and told me what she said.

One of the persons who was supposed to spy on me was coerced by being promised a medication his young child desperately needed and which was not available in Romania. When I realized what was going on [he was supposed to date me, which was completely out of character for that dedicated family man.] I asked the colleague to talk with me somewhere where I was sure no one could hear us, I asked him what was going on, and once I learned the truth, with the help of my in-laws, I obtained the much-needed medication for his child. I never told my in-laws how I found out this man needed the medication.

Another person, who happened to be my technician, was constantly asking me questions about what I was hearing from my husband, in case there were people verbally carrying information between us. I always replied with the content of the letters I was receiving, knowing that the content was already known to authorities.

Working in advanced technology, we also had a person overseeing our activities from a security point of view. I was seated in an area that was clearly visible from his desk. I always made sure that everything I was reading or working on was visible and never showed any interest in finding out anything further about the design that I originally started. Before leaving, this latter person took me aside and told me that my behavior was very wise and congratulated me for it, wishing me good luck in my future endeavors!

Years later, after the fall of the communist regime, I asked my former technician why she spied on me and I shared that she was quite obvious in her questioning. That is when I found out that she intentionally did the obvious questioning, so I knew what to tell her, and she would have safe information to forward to her bosses. She also shared that she decided to report on me because she figured if somebody else would do it, they might not be as kind to me... I am deeply grateful to her.

Finally, after two and a half years, my son and I were able to join Peter. By then I was exhausted. I was also fearful that, even at the last minute, the Romanian government might revoke my passport. I found out only later that the reason I was let go was that the head of Jewish organizations in the U.S. had put me on the list of people that had to be let go in order for Romania to get the Most Favored Nation[26] (MFN)

---

[26] "Most favored nation" (MFN) is a status or level of treatment accorded by one state to another in international trade. The term means the country which is the recipient of this treatment must nominally receive equal trade advantages as the most favored nation by the country granting such treatment. Trade advantages include low tariffs or high import quotas. [Wikipedia.org] This was very important for Romania at the time as exporting to the U.S.A. in favorable conditions meant paying off the foreign debt much faster.

status[27]. No wonder I received the approval to leave the country with the condition that I had to be on the plane to Israel in three weeks. This fast departure caused further problems for us as, once landed in Israel, the authorities there were suspicious of me suddenly being let go from Romania, without Israeli intervention or payment[28].

As soon as I arrived in Israel with my son, I had another shock: Peter told me right away that given that his friend left Israel, he no longer wanted to stay, and we would have to move again. He also told me that he was unemployed during his time in Israel and he got a job only two weeks before my arrival, a job that was paying very little – my husband's salary was less than the car allowance his boss was receiving. Other shocking news was that I had little chance of finding a job, despite my qualifications. This was quite upsetting for me, since I was looking forward to finally settling down and having a peaceful life.

---

[27] This happened just by chance, after everybody else refused to help me and even being tricked by the Romanian government to submit a request for pardon for my husband only to be told after that I had to wait until the government decided on the pardon, because I submitted the request. My husband had a lawsuit against him for defecting, and he got six years in prison and another 2 years of being stripped of citizenship. He never went to prison as he was out of the country.

[28] There was a widely circulating story that Jewish people had to be bought by Israel in order to be allowed to leave.

The first three weeks after my arrival I slept most of the time. My mind literally shut down as it tried to recover from the years of stress. We were staying with my uncle in a wonderful kibbutz[29], where my son had a great time.

After three weeks, Peter had to go for his military service in the Israeli army and I started a Hebrew language school.

While Peter was doing his military service, I decided to do everything possible to prove to him that I can get employment in my field. I went to quite a few interviews, but whatever I did, I could not get a job. I was even examined by a panel of professors to asses if my Ph.D. studies were valid, only to find out, after a full day of questioning, that in fact the professors wanted information about the level of Ph.D. degrees in Romania and the whole exercise had no connection with my possible employment.

---

[29] A kibbutz is a collective community in Israel that was traditionally based on agriculture. Today, farming has been partly supplanted by other economic branches, including industrial plants and high-tech enterprises. Kibbutzim began as utopian communities, a combination of socialism and Zionism. In recent decades, some kibbutzim have been privatized and changes have been made in the communal lifestyle. In 2010, there were 270 kibbutzim in Israel. Their factories and farms account for 9% of Israel's industrial output, worth US$8 billion, and 40% of its agricultural output, which is worth more than $1.7 billion. (English Dictionary in Word)

Slowly we pieced together the truth: my coming to Israel so suddenly, Peter getting into altercations with the person in charge of Romanian immigration, my parents still being in Romania. Hence I was considered a security risk, which contributed to my not finding a job.

It was a real miracle that I was eventually offered a job in my profession on a project not connected with military technology. It was through a kind person who studied engineering at the same school I did and with the same professors. She knew of a company that was desperately looking for a real computer engineer (the previous one had burnt several boards inside the computer when he touched it without knowing what he was doing), and I ended up getting the job. The pay was very low, but I was happy I was useful and not staying at home. It was not what I dreamt of doing in my professional life. I wanted to be part of the computer revolution, to define the technology. As such, I finally agreed to try to emigrate from Israel, although I had family there and nowhere else in the world, except Romania, to which I would return.

We were accepted by two countries in the same week: Australia and Canada. We had to give them a response in two weeks, so for ten days we kept making lists and reading up on both countries. After the jobhunting experience in Israel and being repeatedly told that my profession was the one we could count on for a good income, we decided to go to Canada. The deciding factor was that Canada had the advantage of being close to the U.S.A., so if I did not find employment in Canada, I could go next door and look for a job. I did not have a similar option in Australia.

Peter used his marketing experience ahead of our arrival in Canada and arranged a tentative interview with a Canadian subsidiary of an American company even before our arrival. Eventually I had the interview soon after our arrival and I was hired. Later I learned that I was hired because my boss wanted to be able to say he had a Ph.D. reporting to him.

I was extremely lucky because soon after that I found employment with a company doing computer design, my dream job.

Peter was not as lucky. While being prepared ahead of time that it would be more difficult to find a job for him, we never expected that his diploma in International Trade from a Romanian well-respected university did not mean much to Canadian employers. It took him eight months to land a job which he loved.

We settled and bought a townhouse. The economy in Canada went through a very rough time and at one point the mortgage rates, which changed every year, shot up to 24% and higher. It was very difficult for us, but we made it. In the meantime, my workplace wanted me to transfer to the U.S.A. (more about it later), and we eventually moved.

Knowing Peter's difficulties in finding a job in Canada, I had two conditions for my move to the United States: to have a Green Card, for me and Peter, so we could both be legally employed and to have a job waiting for Peter, which I was promised by my future boss. Unfortunately, it took two and a half years for my company to obtain my Green Card and in the meantime the position promised for Peter no longer existed, so once again he was unemployed.

The fact that Peter could not find any job for years made him very depressed and angry. It was very difficult for him to see me working long hours while he was offered only low paying jobs. So, after three years of unemployment and terrible depression, Peter accepted my suggestion to go and learn what he loved since childhood: how to repair cars. A lot of his previous studies were accepted by the school and two years later Peter had an Associate Degree in Automotive Electronics. Despite being recognized by his workplace as an outstanding technician, this did not ensure a permanent job or a decent income for Peter. Several months after he started work, when there was a seasonal layoff, Peter had enough of the automotive adventure and quit the job. This brought on further depression and anger.

Luckily I knew somebody who had a friend in the Canadian company Peter used to work for before we moved, and through the friend's intervention, Peter was invited back to work for the Canadian company. This meant that Peter lived in Canada, while I stayed in the U.S.A. since, by that time, the Canadian branch of the company I worked for was closed.

Eventually, a year later, I was offered a job at a Canadian company. The CEO of the company was somebody I worked with before and who knew my technical abilities. While I voiced my concern that I was getting out of my profession, the CEO insisted he needed fresh eyes to look at his company's development efforts. I decided to accept the job offer so I could keep the family together. Also, by that time, even the American branch of the company I was working for was in trouble.

Moving to Canada again was difficult. Due to the many hardships my husband went through, he was very controlling. I ended up going from a 2200 square foot house to an efficiency apartment because he refused to get anything bigger. Having entered a completely new technical field, I had to study every night for my new job. Because Peter refused to move to a bigger apartment, I had to study in the tiny bathroom as else my husband would get angry that the light disturbed his sleep. For multiple reasons it was a torturous time, which ended in disaster. I was stressed all the time, partly because of the demands of the job, and partly because of Peter's volatile and controlling nature.

Because of the high level of stress I was continuously under, on a business trip I ended up damaging two of the disks in my lower back. I had to fly back heavily sedated with narcotics to control the excruciating pain. By the time the flight arrived in Toronto, I was in a wheelchair and eventually I had emergency back surgery, after having lost all the muscles in both legs.

After surgery, and after I returned to work full time, I was immediately laid off. That was the only time in my forty years of marriage that Peter brought me flowers. I was laughing and crying because it was so absurd.

With the help of another acquaintance from the technical field, I eventually found another job. By that time computers were designed by computers and only a handful of people were doing actual computer design, mainly architecture definition. My know-how came in handy for the auto industry, as I had knowledge in the area of testing complex systems. This meant another separation for Peter and me.

Following an altercation with the owner of the company, Peter lost his job and was employed by a friend, with a very low salary. The job was a godsend in that it gave Peter a purpose to get dressed in the morning and feel useful, thus avoiding the repeat of the deep depression experienced in the U.S.A.

When I moved back to the U.S.A., Peter stayed with his job to avoid being jobless. In a way it was a reprieve for me as I was starting to feel free of the constant fear of Peter's abusive outbursts. I was happier, and I started to recover my self-esteem. I believe Peter thought I was escaping his control, so when he came for his weekend visit, Peter had another angry outburst and walked with me through the walk-in closet doors, stopping when I hit the back wall. His eyes were glazed over by anger[30] and I feared for my life. He even put his hands on my throat trying to strangle me. Luckily, he 'woke up' and stopped in time.

The following week he gave up his job in Toronto and moved to Michigan, without having another job. Eventually, with the help of my kind boss, Peter was

---

[30] Always Peter's outbursts started with the same declaration: "You are just like my mom", followed by a state in which he was transported, no longer seeing me, probably thinking that he was dealing with his mom. I never found out why he had so much pain related to his relationship with his mother.

able to get a part-time job which, after several years, became permanent.

Peter was not happy. He saw me getting ahead in my career while he was working in a job well below his true capabilities. He did not even try to look for anything else, instead he became angrier and angrier taking out his frustration on me by shouting, belittling me, being controlling, and sometimes even physically abusive. He kept telling me I was an unfit wife, stupid and uneducated. His typical comment was that he did not understand 'how somebody can be such a good engineer and, and at the same time, such a stupid wife.' This happened while, in addition to much longer working hours than Peter's, I did the cooking, cleaning, washing, even sewing my dresses (as a creative outlet).

Eventually my self-esteem plummeted, and I no longer believed in myself. I started feeling like a fake because I was constantly told by Peter that I was worthless, stupid, and ugly, so when I was appreciated at work I was afraid that I would be discovered as a fake. Despite my patents, professional awards, and accolades for constantly solving complicated technical problems, I was under constant stress, afraid I would lose my job and with it everything we had. We could not survive much less save for retirement on Peter's salary.

Things became even more difficult when, due to excess weight, Peter ended up having sleep apnea and refused to go to the sleep specialist. He became even more abusive as his brain was oxygen deprived. He would fall asleep at the office, then come home and demand that all the lights in the house be out by 7:30 pm, when he went to bed. I could not walk in the house once he was asleep as he would wake up at the slightest noise and be very angry and shout at me.

I felt trapped. I was completely separated from my family and I did not have friends. Every time I would try to invite somebody for dinner, Peter would practically dismiss them by 9:00 pm, the latest, either going to sleep or starting to yawn at the table.

Eventually I asked one of my doctor friends I worked with to come to our place and convince Peter to have a sleep apnea test. When the test was done, the sleep specialist was surprised that Peter had not had a heart attack, considering the frequent breathing interruptions during the night.

Even after resolving the sleep apnea, things did not get any better in the way Peter was treating me. The mental abuse became constant. I tried not to share with Peter anything about my life or career as it would be immediately used to demean me and show me how bad and worthless I was. I begged Peter to go for counseling, but he refused.

Then one day, he was very close to choking me. It was triggered when I started to change the oil in the lawnmower. He promised to do it week after week, but it was always postponed. I was the one who had to cut the grass, which was already over 10 inches high, so I could no longer wait. He got angry and started shouting at me pushing me into the shelves that lined the back of the garage. I was ashamed as I saw the neighbors looking at us, so I asked Peter to at least quarrel in private. He took me inside and pushed me into the washer/dryer and started choking me while repeating, as he always did when being physically abusive, 'You are just like my mom.' His eyes, as usual, were no longer seeing me, while his hands were tighter and tighter around my neck. I was sure I was going to die. With a last effort, being hardly able to speak, I looked into Peter's eyes and asked him: 'What are you doing? What are you doing?!' Somehow he 'woke up', released his hold on my neck, turned around, and left. As usual, he never asked for forgiveness, in fact he blamed me for what 'I made him do'.

After that, I always had some clothing in my car and a minimum amount of money in the bank so I could escape in case Peter had a life-threatening bout of anger.

Due to the stress I was under at home and at work, where being over fifty, and a woman, was considered kind of an end to one's career prospects, I ended up having a double brain injury – two slip-and-falls on ice on the same day.

That stopped my life in its tracks. Unfortunately, due to the fear of losing my job and as such not having any retirement benefits, I returned to work much too soon after the accident. That made things worse and I ended up not being able to function at all after a while. It took approximately twelve years to start functioning in an acceptable way for everyday survival, but I was never able to function as an engineer again.

After the accident, it was very difficult because Peter now had valid reasons to berate me. I was no longer able to cook, clean, work, or even sort through the mail. Somehow I kept paying the bills, but I got in trouble with the IRS.

Once, in his frustration, Peter told me that he would put me in a loony bin. As, after the accident, my sleep was so deep that I could not hear or feel anything, following Peter's threat I was afraid to fall asleep. I feared that I would wake up in a mental institution. Together with the constant excruciating pain I had, this ended up causing adrenal exhaustion and eventually fibromyalgia.

After Peter went into early retirement things got even worse. He moved very little and his health started to fail, but he still refused to take care of himself, because I asked him to. He was also obsessively telling me how much better his life would have been if he had stayed in Romania. This made him angrier and angrier and more and more controlling.

I begged him again to go for counseling, but his response was that he had no problem and if had some, I should go. Finally, at the end of my wits, I went into counseling. During the very first session I was told there was not much I could do to change things at home.

As a last resort, Johnny and I tried an intervention, but it failed. The morning after the intervention, while our son was still asleep, Peter walked into me full force, while I was balancing myself on my painful leg. I understood then that I had only two options: leave my marriage and try to recover my health and sanity or stay and either end up in a wheelchair or dead as a result of one of Peter's uncontrolled outbursts.

As Peter kept repeating all the time that he wanted me to leave him alone, with my son's help, I moved into a rented apartment. When after four months I asked Peter if that was the life he wanted, he replied that once I was out of the house I was never coming back. That was when I decided, with Peter's consent, to file for divorce after more than forty years of marriage.

Even after separating from Peter and moving into an apartment, I kept hearing his angry shouting and dreaming of being belittled. Later I would find out that I had PTSD as a result of Peter's behavior."

"That had to be very difficult to take for so many years." Isabelle commented. "How do you feel today about what happened with Peter?"

"I am happy to say that, after having a lot of emotional therapy, I was able to forgive Peter for all the abuse I suffered. I feel a deep compassion as I know it cannot be easy for him. I was told by my therapist that it is a high probability that Peter's emotional wounds are so deep that he is much too afraid of touching them by doing any therapy. I only know that somehow his pain is related to his mother and I suspect it might have been her demeaning behavior toward Peter, but I cannot be sure."

"Was there anything good about your marriage that you can remember?" I heard Isabelle's voice in the distance.

"Yes, there is" I replied. "I am first and foremost grateful for having a wonderful son. Also, I will always be grateful to Peter for introducing me to the books of Carlos Castaneda (the trilogy of "The

Teachings of Don Juan") which was my introduction to alternative therapies. Peter also taught me to appreciate history that, according to him, is more interesting than any novel. Because of his behavior, Peter also gave me a better understanding of abuse, thus making it possible for me to help others[31] in similar situations.

Peter and, through Peter, his friend were the drivers behind our leaving Romania. This provided our son a future that would have been impossible had we stayed. It also opened professional opportunities for me that I would not have had if I stayed in Romania."

"Wow, this is quite a story! You had an eventful life. How is your relationship with Peter today?" Isabelle asked me.

"I do not have a relationship. Peter still feels deeply hurt that I left him, so he does not want to keep in touch. I doubt he ever thought seriously about the reasons that drove me to leaving. His comment when I left was that he never thought I would leave him at that point in life ...and I would not have. I was much too brainwashed. I was lucky to have a son who cared enough about me and a wise future daughter-

---

[31] I thought abuse was an isolated thing that happens in poor, uneducated families. I found later that education or financial status had nothing to do with it.

in-law behind him, to help me escape my hell. Without that help I could not have left."

"What are your feelings about everything that happened in your marriage?" asked Isabelle next.

"I feel a deep compassion for Peter. An educated, good-looking man, who had a talent for seeing things clearly in business, he could have had a much more fulfilling life, if not for the emotional scars left by his mother. I never flaunted my achievements and always stressed his, so he would feel better about himself, but it did not help, and I am deeply sorry for that. I was also very much aware that Peter had difficulty expressing and accepting love, so I did my best to offer him unconditional love every way I could, but he told me he was suspicious of people telling him they love him.

I am grateful that I do not have to be afraid of another angry outburst and I no longer hear Peter's shouting. I am also grateful that I was able to forgive him for all the hardship, fear, and suffering. Today Peter is taking better care of his health and I hope he is happier with his life. As far as I can see, he is living the life he always wanted without having me to disturb his peace. I wish him with all my heart only the very best."

"Anything else you feel you need to bring up?" I heard Isabelle asking again.

"No. I think I am done. It is a lot to process and I am exhausted. I want to rest a bit in the garden before coming back."

"Okay. It is your process. Just step through the mirror and onto the gazebo, then take a walk in your garden. Make sure to notice the trees and the flowers, enjoy the abundance and peace of nature, maybe sit for a while next to the lake. This will help you ground yourself. Let me know when you are ready to come back."

"Yes, I am stepping through the mirror and into the gazebo. What a wonderful day. What a relief to be in nature after such a difficult process! I love the flowers, and the trees, and the birds... they make me feel alive again. Only now I realize that going back into my marriage took the joy of life out of me. I do not even know how I lived so many years in that oppressive environment. I guess I kept hoping that if I changed enough, if I did the things Peter wanted, then maybe one day the kind person I knew lived deep inside him would appear and stay for the rest of our lives and we would be happy together. In trying to change my family environment by changing myself I changed so much, I no longer recognized myself, and it was still not enough. I know today, that nothing I could have done would have been enough."

After taking a few deep breaths I opened my eyes.

"Wow! That was quite a trip down memory lane. I really need some rest."

"I agree" said Isabelle, while I was rubbing my eyes. "Are you sure you can safely get home? Maybe you should consider hanging out at a café for a little while so you can drive home safely."

"I will do that. You are right. I feel like a part of me is still processing the memories and is left behind in the garden. I am seriously considering your suggestion of resting at a café before driving home." With that, I stood up and a little unsure on my feet I said goodbye to Isabelle.

"See you next week!" I heard Isabelle say.

I stayed at the corner café for quite some time, still wondering at some "what ifs" and processing all that I went through in my life. After a while, like waking up from a dream, I could finally notice the lights on the street, the soft snow falling on the sidewalk, and I headed home, looking forward to a hot bath and an inviting bed.

Gaining Insight into Being a Partner

Work through this questionnaire for each person who was a girlfriend/ boyfriend/ husband/ wife/ partner for you.

My girlfriend/ boyfriend/ husband/ wife/ partner

………………….. was……………………………………………..

……………………………………………………………………………..

…………………………………………………………………………….

[Fill in the name and general description, like in: "My husband, Alex, who I am married to for over 40 years, is a kind, considerate, loving man."]

The negative memories I have about……………… are:

1. ………………………………………………………………
   ………………………………………………………………
   ………………………………………………………………
2. ………………………………………………………………
   ………………………………………………………………
   ………………………………………………………………
3. ………………………………………………………………
   ………………………………………………………………
   ………………………………………………………………
4. ………………………………………………………………
   ………………………………………………………………

5. ....
....
....
....

Because of the negative experiences I had with.........
I decided:

1. ....
....
....

2. ....
....
....

3. ....
....
....

4. ....
....
....

5. ....
....
....

[For example: because of the verbal abuse I received from my husband, Paul, I had a very low self-esteem and I decided I must be a fake professionally, if people appreciated me so much.]

My positive life decisions as a result of my negative experiences connected with...........................are:

1. ....
   ....
   ....

2. ....
   ....
   ....

3. ....
   ....
   ....

4. ....
   ....
   ....

5. ....
   ....
   ....

[For example: because of the negative experience and resulting low self-esteem, I decided to use my experience to help others in a similar situation...]

The positive memories related to .... are:

1. ....
   ....
   ....

2. ....
   ....
   ....

3. ....
   ....
   ....

4. ....
....
....
5. ....
....
....

Because of the positive experiences I had with.........
I decided:

1. ....
....
....
2. ....
....
....
3. ....
....
....
4. ....
....
....
5. ....
....
....

[For example: because of the knowledge my
husband shared about........ and the enthusiasm he
had for it, I decided to learn more about the that
field.]

The top five blessings that come from my experiences with .... are:

1. ....
   ....
   ....

2. ....
   ....
   ....

3. ....
   ....
   ....

4. ....
   ....
   ....

5. ....
   ....
   ....

[For example: I understood that abuse is much more common inside families than I previously thought; I became aware of the deeply damaging long-term effects of emotional abuse.]

Being a Mother
෬ ෭

"Welcome!" Isabelle greeted me as I entered her office. "Ready for another trip down memory lane, or you need some more time on any of the previous topics?"

"I am ready for the next topic" I replied. "I would like to work today on my experiences as a mother. I wanted to be a mother as long as I can remember. My parents told me that, from an early age, I was taking good care of my dolls. When I finally had a sister, I was elated and I happily gave her all my dolls to destroy. I no longer needed them because I had my own living, breathing child.

When I got married, I could not wait to become a mother and, given the Romanian laws at the time[32]

---

[32] At the time, by governmental decree, every woman in Romania had to have a minimum of four children. This was enforced by the lack of any kind of birth control measures. Later, because of the high rate of illegal abortions, they introduced a rule that every woman had to be examined each month by a doctor at her workplace, to make sure that she did not have an illegal abortion. If a person was found to have done anything to the fetus, both the woman and the person helping her would land in prison! This resulted in many women resorting to very primitive measures of aborting, frequently puncturing their uterus and dying from the hemorrhage.

which required women to have a minimum of four kids, we had a son in a little over a year after we got married. It was a dream come true."

"How did Peter react to you being pregnant and later having a child?" asked Isabelle.

"I think he was scared. Looking back, I think for him marrying was more of a practical decision, and he did not really connect it with childbearing. So, during my pregnancy he usually came home very late at night. He worked in international trade, so he was invited to the dinners which were part of the selling process. He spoke perfect British English, so he was often the translator at those dinners. Maybe being at work so much was a welcomed escape for him."

"And after you gave birth?" enquired Isabelle.

"After I gave birth, Peter became even busier. He was rarely home before Johnny went to bed. He also

---

Because of the drive to pay off the foreign debt, the salaries were very low, and people were practically starving. Only food that was of too low a quality to be exported was given to the Romanian citizens. As an example, both my husband and I were college graduates with the best salaries available at the time and by the end of the month – having only one child – we had to get food supplies from my in-laws as we did not have the money to buy food. In order to get staples such as oil, flour, or cornmeal, I had to take off from work and stay in line with my son, a baby at the time, so we could get one allotment each (1 kg /2.2 lbs of something was the typical allotment). You could not just walk into a food store and buy unlimited quantities.

Being a Mother

began taking French lessons at work. I remember during the time I was home with our son after delivery, Peter asked me to pick him up at work so he could drive his teacher home because she had a painful period. By the time I finished breastfeeding our son, I got into peak traffic, so I was late. As soon as he saw me, Peter berated me in front of his teacher. He was extremely angry that I did not tell him I would be late, but in those times we did not have cell phones, so I had no way of calling once in the car. He reminded me many times of this 'awful behavior'."

"I believe it is time for you to go through your next mirror so we can see your life as a mother and the gift in that experience." Isabelle gently guided me back to the subject at hand. "Close your eyes and take a few deep breaths… Good! Now you find yourself in your enchanted garden, walking around, enjoying the trees, the flowers, the birds, the lake. Are you there?"

"Yes. I love it! It always relaxes me. It is so beautiful." I readily replied.

"Wonderful! Find your gazebo and your next mirror and let me know when you stepped through the mirror." I heard Isabelle in the distance.

"I have just stepped through the mirror. I am so happy! I just gave birth a few hours ago and I am admiring my son. He is so tiny and so perfect. I tell him how glad I am he is mine, how much fun we are going to have together, how much his dad, aunt, and grandparents look forward to meeting him.

Next I see myself, as a true scientist, insisting to get on a scale to find out how much weight I lost through the birthing process. The nurses do not understand why I need to know that, but they indulge me because I had such a difficult birth[33].

My next image is still from the hospital. My beloved cousin, a doctor, is the first to come and visit me. In those times people were not allowed to visit mothers and newborns in the ward, they had to go to a special room several floors down. As I had to be in bed, still recovering from the birthing process, going down was out of the question. To this day I am deeply grateful to my cousin for his visit. He told me he offered his doctor's badge to Peter so he could visit me (they looked very much the same in pictures), but

---

[33] As my mother would find out later, through a careless comment from the attending doctor, both Johnny and I nearly died during the birthing process. The normal birthing process was stopped, because the doctor did not want to come to the hospital that night. Ten days later, Johnny's heartbeat was faint and mine was irregular, so I was hospitalized. The doctor tried unsuccessfully every possible method to induce the birth. In the end, a very large nurse pushed the baby out by compressing my belly. I was lucky I went through the birthing process without making a sound, despite not having any anesthetic. According to the attending physician, it saved both our lives.

Peter refused for fear they would pull him into some doctoring discussion.

The next image is of us at my parents' home. We stayed there the first two weeks. Johnny slept on a sofa chair, while we took over my parents' bed. In those times we did not have disposable diapers, so I had to wash and boil the diapers every day in a large pot, which was impossible for me to lift right after the birth. I can still remember the smell of diapers boiling in soap and bicarbonate of soda.

From that time, I also remember my mother's concern when I wanted to name our son after my father. In European Jewish tradition one does not name somebody after a living person[34], so she was concerned something terrible would happen to my dad, who was away on a business trip. My in-laws insisted on naming our son after one of them but, after the difficult thirty-two-hours birth, they let me name our son whatever I wanted, they were happy we were alive.

My father was very proud I named my son after him. He kept calling Johnny 'my namesake' instead of his name. My mother also relented once dad was safely home.

---

[34] There is no such restriction in Sephardi Jewish tradition.

Next I see my father-in-law visiting. He was amused that Peter and I was were finally playing 'house' for real. My father-in-law loved children. He would have liked very much for us to have more. Both he and my father were totally taken by the new male in the family.

I can see now in rapid succession our Sunday ritual, when Peter and Johnny would be in bed while I would prepare the traditional cocoa. Then the summer vacations with my sister at the seashore. I can see the day Johnny, my father-in-law, and I took Peter to the airport for his three months of marketing studies in England, which ended up being two and a half years of separation for the two of us, and many more years of separation from his parents.

I can see my time with my son after Peter's defection. Johnny's discovery of the world around him was a permanent highlight of my days. He was curious as he was handy, so my father enjoyed teaching him how to assemble stuff and build gadgets they enjoyed. My father was in love with that little smart, wide-eyed kid, who was full of life and possibilities.

My mother helped me educate my son. My sister loved playing with Johnny, and even took him on her dates as a safety net, as my son would later tell me.

We were very proud of Johnny's development. Once he started kindergarten, he showed his budding leadership qualities. His teachers told me he had a special talent to do with the kids what the teachers wanted: get them in line, break up fights, or share his knowledge. This talent of influencing people would serve him well later in life, in his endeavors as a business owner.

Once it was discovered that Peter defected, we were summoned to Peter's uncle who was the one to receive the letter telling about the defection. He did not know that I knew of Peter's plans, but he told me – while his wife was playing with Johnny – that I could be in prison if they ever found out I knew. It was kind of him to warn me.

Next I see Johnny staying with my parents. No one knew what would happen to me as a result of Peter's defection, so we decided it was safer for Johnny if he were not at home with me. I visited him every day after work. I usually had dinner at my parents as by the time I would get home it was late at night. That stopped the day I was told that I sat down at the table like a 'cow expecting to be fed'! I still visited, but pretended to have already had my dinner, even though, due to my strained financial situation, many times I could afford only one meal a day. My income had gone down and I had to buy back my own furniture as the government claimed it as its right because of Peter's defection. My in-laws gave me money to cover the furniture payments, but I decided to give the money to my parents for my son's care, so they would not have financial hardships caring for Johnny. I was immensely grateful Johnny was in a loving, caring environment.

Johnny developed very nicely, nurtured with lots of love. There were some hiccups though. I remember a time when I was trying to teach my son addition. I tried apples, nuts, matches (yes, we still had matches), but nothing. Then I remembered that every morning I was teaching Johnny how to pay for the tram tickets, so I gave him some singles. He immediately started adding without any problems. I believe in Johnny's mind, counting money was a useful pursuit.

Next I see the day I was called by Johnny's kindergarten teacher because he beat up a child, something totally out of character. The teacher was a friend of mine, and when we pieced together the events, we found that the child told Johnny that his father was waiting to pick him up from kindergarten. In fact, it was my own father (who looked always much younger than his age), so Johnny was deeply disappointed and took out his frustration on the boy. It was up to me to explain to Johnny that he could not expect to see his father for a long time as he was far away, and we could not go to visit him either.

After some inklings that something was amiss while my son was at my parents, I decided I would do whatever I could to bring him back to live with me. I had to paint my apartment, which was my parents' condition for allowing me to take Johnny home. After painting, the apartment looked awful[35], but it was clean.

After two and a half years of separation, we finally got the approval to leave. As it was a miracle my son was kept in the kindergarten after Peter's defection, I told Johnny the good news that we would see his dad again, but I warned him he should not tell anyone. He asked me if it was okay to tell his beloved teacher (who was my friend) and I agreed. So, in the afternoon, when his teacher was supposed to come in, Johnny could not fall asleep. Immediately after the change of shift, my friend made her usual rounds. As soon as she came into Johnny's room, my son jumped up and down on his bed and in a room full of sleeping kids started shouting: 'We have the passport! We have the passport! We are going to my daddy!' He was immediately pulled out of the room. Luckily Johnny was able to be with his kindergarten friends until the day we left the country.

Once I knew for sure that we had the visa and the airplane ticket was safely in my pocket, after a short

---

[35] We did not have rollers or formulas for exact dilution of the paint, so my ceilings and walls were all streaked.

trip with my parents, Johnny and I stayed for a week in the Romanian mountains. We no longer had a place to live, so it was a pleasant ending after some tough times. I used this opportunity to convince Johnny to stop sucking his thumb. I told him, if he stopped sucking his thumb, we were going to see his dad in ten days, and I counted them on his fingers. Johnny never sucked his thumb again. I could see him, for a couple of days, start to raise his thumb to his mouth and stop halfway. I was proud of Johnny's strength while my heart was breaking as I thought how difficult it had to be for him to do it."

"How was the meeting with Peter? Did Johnny recognize him?" I heard Isabelle's voice.

"I made sure to prepare Johnny for the meeting." I replied. "After the incident when Johnny beat up his kindergarten friend, I put away all of Peter's pictures and we made sure not to talk about him in front of Johnny. I also asked my in-laws not to remind Johnny of his father, not to create unnecessary pain. They were really understanding, and I was grateful for that. Once the shock of losing their son dulled a bit, my in-laws would have done anything to protect Johnny in any way possible.

Once I knew that we were leaving for sure, I took out Peter's photos and started telling stories about him. I continued this while Johnny and I were together in the mountains. I also prepared Johnny for having to leave his beloved grandparents and aunt behind encouraging him to be nice and loving to everyone, to ease the separation. Johnny, only five years old, somehow understood and was very kind to everyone.

When we arrived in Israel, we had to have our papers checked, which took some time. I had an uncle who was well known, even beyond his kibbutz, as a very loving man. He was able to get inside the secure area with Peter, and they took care of Johnny while I took care of the paperwork. In the beginning Johnny was frightened of the tall, powerful-looking man in front of him, but then I reminded him of the pictures in which he saw Peter's curly hair and I offered him to climb up on Peter's shoulders. (He loved being carried by my father that way.) Once up on Peter's shoulders Johnny was happy, and father and son were great friends again.

My family showered a lot of love on Johnny, so he felt immediately at home. Soon he was speaking Hebrew like a native. He did not like that his father was away for military service, but he enjoyed playing with Peter's stuff when he was home on furlough.

We also traveled from time to time to job interviews and visited relatives in our travels. Johnny loved to be at my uncle's kibbutz. My uncle would proudly show him off and take him to the swimming pool, where Johnny would stay in the water for hours. I think he enjoyed the experience and the love around him, so it was not easy when we moved again, this time to a much colder climate, in December of 1978, during one of the coldest winters on record..

Once in our Canadian hotel room, I could see Johnny's excitement when we found cartoons on the TV. We both stayed up all night watching them and laughing. Johnny was delighted when the next day we went out and, using the last of our money, we bought two submarine sandwiches[36]. He ate a whole one all by himself, delighted to have so many cold cuts in a single seating.

Next I remember Johnny's joy after he spent the day with our new friend Mark[37] while we were looking for an apartment. Mark spoke Italian, Johnny Romanian, and they had a great time. They remained fast friends while Mark was alive.

I also remember Johnny's excitement when we moved to our place and when he would tell me about his school. He loved Canada so much, only one month after arriving in Canada, he would claim he was born there and never lived anywhere else.

---

[36] The submarine sandwiches are very big and are made with a long bread overstuffed with cold cuts.

[37] He was the uncle of my best friend from Israel. Much older than us, already retired, he could relate to each of us at our level.

It was wonderful watching Johnny grow, make friends, and learn new things. I was discovering the world again through his eyes, caught up in his enthusiasm. Minor things that I did not even notice were something to be studied, enjoyed, or both. He made friends among the smart kids who were avidly learning new things. Johnny had mainly friends who were immigrants like him: from India, from Russia, from Japan. He was interested in stories about those countries as well as readily sharing whatever he knew, be it information that added to their studies or his life experience.

I remember once, after introducing Johnny to a wonderful book called 'What Is Happening to Me',[38] when his friends came over, Johnny and his friends went upstairs to his room, as usual. What was unusual was the deep silence that every parent knows typically spells trouble with kids. So, I went upstairs and opened the door to Johnny's bedroom. I found his friends sitting on the floor in a semicircle, while Johnny was standing and explaining the book. I asked Johnny to come talk with me and I explained to him that it was best to stop the meeting since other parents would probably want to have the opportunity to share the information with their kids. Johnny happily replied: 'It is okay mom; I am done anyway. Can I come to you if we have any

---

[38] This book, which is in print for a long time, is a very simple sex education book for very young children.

questions?' I was surprised and I replied: 'Yes, of course.' Ten or fifteen minutes later I had quite a few questions from the children, one was: 'Is it true that, if a woman stands on her head after making love, she would not get pregnant?'... He was only eight years old.

Johnny was a responsible kid. Peter went to the office late, after Johnny left for school. Nobody was home when Johnny returned, so he had the house key, and he always came home directly from school and waited for me to come home an hour later. I would give him something to snack on, then we would discuss his day at school. It was a pleasant routine, we both enjoyed. One day when Johnny came home from school, he sat me down and, with a very serious face, asked me if I knew what f**k meant. After I recovered from the shock, I replied, 'Sorry, I don't know. Do you?' At this my son replied: 'I have no idea, but I know if somebody tells you that, you should NOT say thank you.'

Drugs were not as big a problem in Canada as they were in the U.S.A., but there were still people pushing drugs to the kids. I was terrified by it, so we discussed that topic too, after we watched a serial on Public TV about it. Luckily Johnny never got involved with drugs.

Eventually we moved into a townhome. I remember that some of Johnny's classmates would not associate with kids, unless they lived in a home, so we did our best to get into one as soon as we could. Peter even got a loan against his future earnings in order to have the amount needed for the down payment. I found out later that 'being in a house' was not enough, one had to be in the right house to be part of the group. We explained to Johnny that the real value is not in what house one lives in but in the love that is in that home and that, for his future, the size of the house had no bearing, but knowledge had. So, using some math books sent by my parents from Romania we started teaching Johnny more advanced math than what he was learning in school. He liked it and he became very good at it. Unfortunately, being a very sensitive child and the other children being aware of this, he was frequently taunted as a brownnoser the pain of which deeply etched in his memory.

Johnny's love of mathematics and reading qualified him for an admission test to a gifted children's school associated with Toronto University. He took the exam, but by the time the results came in, we were already transferred to the United States. This started a new chapter in all our lives. For Johnny it meant having some amazing professors, as he was immediately placed in the advanced program, corresponding to the Toronto gifted program.

I remember Johnny coming home from school his first week and telling me: 'Mom, this school provides everything: drugs, sex, and top-notch learning.' 'So, what do you choose?' I asked him. After waiting for a few seconds, Johnny winked and replied: 'Learning, of course'... and he took fully advantage of the learning opportunities.

In Minnesota most of the population was descended from Nordic or German stock, so Johnny – as an East European – stood out. He was bullied to the level of getting sick, at which point his homeroom teacher intervened, having a discussion with the class while Johnny was home. He was never bullied again.

Unfortunately, a combination of moving around so much, Peter's outbursts (he was unemployed at the time), and the bullying at school, resulted in Johnny being diagnosed with Cushing disease, a tumor on his adrenals. His cortisol was highly elevated, and his skin was gray with the under-arm skin parting. After a 24-hour urine test, Johnny was scheduled for a kidney x-ray. Luckily, using my healing abilities, by the time of the x-ray appointment Johnny had recovered and no tumor was found during the test. Our family doctor repeated the urine test, and that was normal too.

Slowly Johnny developed a circle of friends, youngsters who liked learning. Their favorite pastime was playing strategy games. It was delightful watching the seriousness of their play.

As much as I tried to shield my son from the stress of Peter not having a job, I am sure Johnny felt it too. He was a good student, but never fully acknowledged his own strengths. Johnny received recognition for his math and physics accomplishments, as well as for his knowledge of Latin. At home he studied French, which he perfected during a Rotary-organized student exchange in Belgium.

It was hard for me to let Johnny go away to Europe for nine months and, at the same time, I was happy for the opportunity he had to learn about other cultures and how to adapt to an environment outside his family.

During his time in Europe, Johnny again proved himself an able leader, organizing trips around Europe for himself and his fellow Rotary friends. The trip to Belgium would also mark the beginning of Johnny leaving home. Once he got back from Belgium, he went away to study at Stanford.

To prove to Johnny how good he really was, I encouraged him to apply to all the universities he thought he wanted to attend but was convinced he would not be accepted. He was accepted by all eight of the universities to which he applied. He had a difficult time deciding which one to attend, finally settling on Berkley, Stanford, or MIT. Berkley offered him scholarship, but no deferral, while the latter two were willing to defer him for the year spent in Europe. The decision to attend Stanford was made after a discussion with a wonderful boss of mine, who was teaching at both institutions. Johnny never regretted the decision to attend Stanford, even if it was difficult at times. At Stanford the students were the best of the best from all over the country, so it was much more difficult to be one of the top students, but Johnny was still one of the top ones.

I was highly honored that Johnny kept in close contact with us while he was a student. He valued our opinion and we tried to support him as best we could, taking his late-night calls, even when they were in the early morning. I remember a few times when he thought he was calling at 8:00 pm, when in fact it was 2:00 am on the East Coast. ...I was still took his calls and patiently discussed whatever the topic. His trust meant more to me than a few hours of sleep.

Once in the work force, Johnny built companies with his Stanford friends. He enjoyed the process and learned a lot from it, preparing him for the company he eventually built with his wife.

After a couple of long-term relationships, a smart, beautiful Brazilian woman stole his heart for good.

Seeing his happiness in his marriage, his success in building his businesses, and how good a father he is, fills my heart with pride and my life with joy.

I still think that being a mother, and now a grandmother, is the most rewarding experience of all. There were and still are times when I worry about him and his family or I am hurt by some things that happen, but all the worry and pain melts away in the moments of joy they bring into my life."

"I see you did not have any negative experiences with your son, but do you have any lessons that you learned? What was the gift in being a mother?" I heard Isabelle asking.

"I saw Heaven in the eyes of my newborn, I learned to appreciate the world's beauty at a level that adults can no longer see, I experienced the deepest unconditional love, and now the joys of being a grandmother. I would never exchange them for anything in the world!"

"Is there anything else you would like to look at in this session?"

"No, I believe I am just about ready to leave my garden."

"Then step through the mirror and walk in your garden, so you can come back again." Isabelle directed me.

As I walked through my imaginary garden I felt light, full of joy, and the colors of the flowers seemed brighter. Going through my experiences as a mother recharged me, giving me a feeling of quiet satisfaction.

Once back, I felt happy, ready to dance. Yes, I did have my life's dream come true by having a son. My life was not lived in vain.

I left Isabelle's office, after agreeing to see her the following week, and I went home to enjoy quietly the wonderful glow left by my session with Isabelle.

Gaining Insight into Being a Parent

Work through this questionnaire for each one of your children. If you did not have any children, but you happened to be the caretaker for younger siblings, or other people's children, do the exercise for those too.

.... was...

....

....

[Fill in the name of the person and a general description, such as: "My son Ed, who is my youngest, gave me a lot of problems."]

The negative memories I have about.................. are:

1 ....
   ....
   ....
2. ....
   ....
   ....
3. ....
   ....
   ....
4. ....
   ....

....

5. ....

....

....

Because of the negative experiences I had with.........
I decided:

1. ....

....

....

2. ....

....

....

3. ....

....

....

4. ....

....

....

5. ....

....

....

[For example: because of the negative experiences I
had with Ed, I decided not to have any more kids.]

My positive life decisions as a result of my negative
experiences connected with...........................are:

1. ....

....
....
2. ....
....
....
3. ....
....
....
4. ....
....
....
5. ....
....
....

[For example: because of the negative experiences with Ed, I decided to start a support group for parents in similar situations as mine. This support group ended up giving me tools to better deal with my own children.)

The positive memories related to .... are:

1. ....
....
....
2. ....
....
....
3. ....
....

4. ....
....
....

5. ....
....
....

Because of the positive experiences I had with.........
I decided:

1. ....
....
....

2. ....
....
....

3. ....
....
....

4. ....
....
....

5. ....
....
....

[For example: because of the positive results I had
with the support group I decided to transform it into
a worldwide organization.]

The top five blessings that come from my experiences with ……………. are:

1. ……………………………………………………………………
……………………………………………………………………
……………………………………………………………………
2. ……………………………………………………………………
……………………………………………………………………
……………………………………………………………………
3. ……………………………………………………………………
……………………………………………………………………
……………………………………………………………………
4. ……………………………………………………………………
……………………………………………………………………
……………………………………………………………………
5. ……………………………………………………………………
……………………………………………………………………
……………………………………………………………………

[For example: I understood that I was not alone; I made a lot of friends; I have today an awesome support system, etc.]

Being a Professional
CঙEO

"Are you ready to step through the last mirror or do you feel we need to go back and explore some more the previous ones?" Isabelle asked me as soon as I stepped into her office.

"I believe I am ready for the last one," I replied, settling on the couch.

"How did you feel after the last the session?" Isabelle asked.

"Absolutely wonderful. I felt so energized and happy, I decided to stay up for a while just to prolong the enjoyment of that feeling. Finally, I had something in my life that gave me more satisfaction than pain and taught me through positive experiences. Believe me, after the rest of the sessions, it was a welcomed respite."

"Do you need anything before we start? Do we need to discuss anything?"

"No, I believe I am ready for the next trip."

"You know the process. Just settle in, take deep breaths, find your enchanted garden, and walk in it to fully relax. Let me know when you are ready to head to the gazebo."

"Oh, I love walking in my garden! It is so colorful. Having the opportunity to experience the garden, when outside is snow and sleet, is truly wonderful. Can I take a bit of time to enjoy it?"

"It is your session, so you are in command. Take your time. Just tell me when you are ready to step through the last mirror."

I wondered through my imaginary garden taking in the sight of the brightly colored flowers, the chirping of the birds, and the smell of the lake nearby. I wanted to remember it all when done with the sessions. Reluctantly, I headed for the gazebo so I could start my last trip.

"I am ready to climb the steps to the gazebo... I am doing it... I am in front of the mirrors... I am stepping through the one with the 'Being a Professional' sign above it."

"Good! Now we can begin our work." I heard Isabelle's voice sounding as if she was far away. "What is the most important thing that you remember about your profession?"

"I remember how happy and exhilarated I was every time I had to solve some complicated engineering problem. At one point of my career they called me Mikey[39] because I was

---

[39] Mikey was the youngest kid in a TV advertisement, in which the older ones refused to try a new cereal, so they gave it to Mikey to try. Once they saw Mikey liked it, the older ones ate it too.

Being a Professional

assigned all the problems others refused to get their teeth into for fear of failing."

"How did you get into your profession? Engineering was not a field women of your generation would choose."

"I wanted first to be a pilot, but I had to give up on that idea when I found out they would not accept women. My next dream profession was nuclear physicist, as I perceived the opportunities for invention in that field. That idea was abandoned too, when I learned that once people started to work at the nuclear reactor, they could no longer have kids. This interfered with my dream of being a mother. For a while I considered becoming a doctor, as I had a pretty good intuition of what to do when members of my family got sick. I loved taking care of them and making them feel better[40]. That idea was abandoned too, when I was told about the 'trial by fire' of the anatomical dissections.

Engineering was the last one I considered because I liked to tinker with stuff. I loved repairing things when they broke. My first memory of repairing something by myself was standing on a kitchen chair and repairing a fuse. In those days, it was a fairly dangerous enterprise, as you had to wrap a certain number of thin wires around the ceramic fuse, then screw the fuse head back on. One could easily get electrocuted, if one touched the wires at the end of the

---

[40] My father inspired me in this as he had the same capability. Later in life I found out that anyone can do it, if the person is honestly interested in helping people.

process. I was sure I could do it safely as I watched my father doing it many times. I also asked questions about the number of wires required, and I was warned about the dangers of electrocuting myself. I was very young, maybe eight years old, when I pulled one of the kitchen chairs close to the fuse box, climbed on it unscrewed the ceramic fuse top, carefully removed the burnt wires, counted them, and then replaced them.

I was very proud of my handiwork once the fuse was back in its place. Just then, my dad opened the door. He came home earlier than usual as he had to go back to work later for a meeting. When he saw what I did, he asked me first if I remembered that he forbade me to repair any electrical stuff. I told him I remembered, but I wanted to surprise him. Very calmly, my dad asked me to get off the chair, get a wet cloth, take off my shoes, then climb back up the chair. I was quite surprised he was not upset. Then he told me, to my utter surprise, to put the wet cloth under my right foot, then show him my right hand. 'Okay', he said, 'now touch the fuse wire with your right hand.' As one could expect, I was zapped by electricity. 'Now you understand why I told you not to touch anything electrical?' my father asked. 'Yes, I do' I answered sheepishly, 'but why all this setup with the wet cloth and the insistence of having it under my right foot and touching the fuse with the right hand?' My dad proceeded to explain that wet things are better electricity conductors and he insisted the electricity go through the right side of my body, to avoid directing it through my heart. I never forgot the lesson in how to deal with electricity safely. After a few fuse repairs under my father's supervision, I was allowed to do them by myself.

By the age of twelve I was doing most of the repairs not requiring heavy lifting. I was having lots of fun with them while dad was bragging about it to anyone willing to listen.

It was only natural to head for engineering, but which branch? One of my father's friends was among the first automation engineers in the country. His house had shutters and curtains opening at the push of a button. I loved it, so I decided that I was going to learn that profession and build myself a home with lots and lots of automation in it.[41] Automation engineering was a fairly new field at the time and, once in that field of study, I was offered the opportunity to go into a newly developing field: that of computers. It would require me to take additional courses, but I was excited about it.

When I had to choose the topic for my Master of Science thesis, I selected a computer design that used circuits modeling the neural cells, another topic of interest of mine. I was mesmerized by the way our brain works and voraciously read anything I could find about it. In the process of preparing my thesis I attended my first scientific

---

[41] The house with "lots and lots of automation in it" was going to have trap doors hiding furniture that would open and replace the existing furniture with a different set. Due to the complexity of building such a house and the cost involved, it remains a dream to this day.

conferences. I did it so I would get over my fear of public speaking.

My thesis was well received, and I was invited by my professor to continue the work through to a Ph.D. I was excited to have the opportunity to continue my work with such a distinguished person[42], so I gladly accepted.

I took my Ph.D. admission exam when I was six months pregnant and started my Ph.D. studies with a four months old baby. It was not easy by any means especially since, at that time, I was also working full time on the design of the first commercial computer in Romania's history. I was lucky I could survive on very little sleep, so I was able to do it all. The work on the computer design gave me the opportunity to be responsible for the floating-point unit[43], as we were all learning a new field. My part of the design was delivered on time and no one could ever find any design errors in my floating point unit. I also passed my Ph.D. prerequisite exams with flying colors and wrote the necessary papers. My thesis was warmly received by the committee of professors... then my husband defected, and my career got tanked. I was no longer allowed to even look at my previous work for the next generation of computers, being relegated to the work of a technical translator until the day I was finally able to leave the country and join my husband.

---

[42] My professor was internationally known for his groundbreaking work in electrical distribution automation using computers.
[43] The part of the computer that enables it to work with very large numbers.

My Ph.D. advisor tried to push through the public defense of my thesis, the last step in my Ph.D. program, but he was advised to 'stop trying, if he valued his health', euphemism for 'if you don't want to go to jail, or worse, you will stop trying to help the wife of a defector.'

Despite the abrupt end of my Romanian career, I have fond memories of the design I was involved in and the people I worked with.

The next stage of my career was dedicated to installing a computer-driven traffic control system in downtown Tel-Aviv. It was difficult because they did not have experience working with a woman engineer, and saw me as some helpless housewife, who just happened to have an engineering diploma. Luckily I was saved by a German technician from Siemens who vouched for my technical abilities which surpassed his. That solved my issues with the owner, but the line workers were something else. Hired because I spoke English, the workers assumed I did not know Hebrew, so all day long they were making comments about me such as 'instead of trying to boss us around, you should be home washing your husband's underwear and cooking him dinner'. I just listened and ignored their remarks until the day they started destroying the underground sensor network to sabotage me. I told them to stand aside, took the phone connecting us to the people in the field, and started reconnecting the wires. They were shocked: the 'housewife' knew how to do their job and she could even solder. The latter for some reason freaked them out and they started shouting that I was going to burn myself and the owner will accuse them of not doing their job. I calmly let them know that I was soldering and working with electrical circuits since the age of twelve, and if they wanted their job, they needed to stop the sabotage, or I was going to tell the company owner what they were doing. The company owner was not known as being a nice man, so no one wanted to get on his bad side.

After that day, I never had any problems with the workers, in fact I even acquired a special position in their hierarchy as they were bragging about having a woman project leader who knew how to do 'manly' work.

The next stage of my profession proved to be even more interesting. I was fortunate enough to be involved in yet another technology revolution: the definition of integrated technology design. It was wonderful to be again in an environment where I could create new ways of designing computers, defining tools to design those computers and finding new ways to work with the technology. In order to acquaint myself with the new technology trends, I even built a computer in my basement. It was running the Microsoft operating system and it had BASIC, a very easy programming language. The latter was used by my son in junior high to do some very simple programming and by my husband to do assembly level programming for his Associate Automotive Engineering studies."

"How was being a woman in a man's world, as I suppose in those times, even in Canada, there were not many women in your profession?" Isabelle asked me.

"In Romania I was easily accepted as part of the team, as long as I could put up with the extra long hours required by the design. I was readily entrusted with designing a whole complex part of the computer by myself. I received some help only when it came to physically verifying the computer we designed. I fondly remember the surprise and appreciation from my colleagues when they could never find any errors in my design, as in those days every piece of the design was verified by hand. This meant that the designer himself had to come up with the right test cases for his part and then apply them to the design drawings one at a time. It was boring work that required long stretches of time of intense focus exclusively on the design, so most of us were not very fond of the process.

In Canada, after the first reaction of not knowing what to expect from me or how to treat me, I was accepted as a member of the team. I was the first female engineer in the company, and I am proud to say that they must have liked having one, because after some time, they hired some more young female engineers. As I had experience mentoring young engineers, I became the protector and guide for these women, especially teaching them the work/home balance, which was the most difficult to accomplish. They stayed, and 'women engineers' became just 'engineers', like everybody else, and after some time, we even got paid on par with our male counterparts.

The interview for my Canadian design position took a whole day and then I was called again for additional interviewing, before I was hired. When I went to interview for the American branch, they no longer wanted to see my diplomas and told me they did not need to interview me as they saw my work. In fact, instead of the interview I was shown several job opportunities and allowed to speak with people in different groups that needed my expertise. This was a pleasant surprise for me. Once hired, I always felt I was a full-fledged member of the team, and being a woman was never an issue.

The best years and perhaps the most creative of my career were spent in defining the integrated technology and the tools to design it with, and later educating people from other companies on how to use the new technology correctly. The company was a true engineering company, allowing us to go as far out on a limb as we wanted, if we could prove the economic benefit of our ideas. At one point I was even given five research engineers to implement an idea I had for improving design turnaround. We were able to design an expert system that mimicked my work as a designer, and produced in five to ten minutes the results I, as an expert, needed three weeks to obtain.

Unfortunately, due to the lack of vision on the part of the company owners, they missed an important opportunity to commercialize the technology we developed, and the company ran into increasingly worse financial troubles, until it completely disappeared. The worst for me came the day all the people in Advanced Research were laid off. I knew each one of them and the families of most. They were talented, smart, hard-working people, who had families to feed. The layoffs had a significant effect on me. I could no longer stay with a company that treated its precious resources that way.

I nearly got hired by IBM, being offered to name my salary, but judging from the way the management worked, building local fiefdoms, I had an inkling the company was in trouble. Sure enough, a few months later over sixteen thousand people were let go, and most probably I would have been one of them, had I accepted the job offer.

I ended up back in Canada, starting one of the most difficult chapters of my career as an engineer. The job was difficult, not only because I was in a totally different engineering field, but mostly because of taking a job that my direct boss wanted for one of his friends. To top it off, I was again the only woman engineer in the company and I had to fight yet again all the stereotypes associated with it. It did not help that the CEO, who brought me into the company, fell in love with his secretary and no longer was interested in the company or in coaching me. I was at the mercy of a man who did not want me and who derived great pleasure from putting me down every chance he got. The stress affected me deeply, and I ended up with several burst disks in my back, that required surgery. The company was in financial trouble, as soon as I returned from medical leave, I was immediately laid off together with all my research team. This was the most painful chapter in my career, but I still remember some exceptional people I met there.

My next job was highly satisfying from a technical point of view. I had the opportunity to be on the leading edge of technology development, this time by defining a new approach to testing car electronics. By that time cars and trucks were being built with lots of microcomputers that controlled everything from window movement, to vehicle speed, combustion, and brakes. The industry needed a way to simplify testing while at the same time make it more effective, since people's lives depended on it.

I remember my first walk-through after I was hired. I asked how the engineers knew that the electronics would work when placed in the car. The reply shocked me: 'We just pray that it does.' I knew I had my work cut out for me.

I met a lot of talented engineers at that company and had some projects that required the collaboration of people from different backgrounds: British, German, and North American. My background as an immigrant served me well, and I was able to teach people to appreciate the strengths that others had, while also sharing their own strengths.

Yes, I was able to improve the testing and again people trusted me as an engineer. I loved going to work every day to meet the new technical challenges, but I was not very happy because my career advancement was limited once I turned fifty. If men have problems once they reach a certain age, the problem is much worse for women. It is a more pervasive image of women being 'aged'.

After the promise of a promotion, when the rug was pulled from under me several times, I decided to focus on doing what I loved and no longer care about the political games played by some. I took daring technical assignments, re-trained young engineers when their qualifications were no longer needed by the company, and I readily taught my newly developed design and test techniques to young people who left to promote them in other parts of the company. I loved being the incubator for new technical thinking.

Unfortunately, at some point the age discrimination became toxic: I was repeatedly asked to develop new presentations based on my original work, then present them to a younger engineer, a favorite of my boss, who would in turn present the work as their own at vice-president level.[44] This combined with very long working hours, sometimes starting at 4:00 am, ended my career, following a double traumatic brain injury due to slip-and-fall on ice.

I still miss the excitement of engineering discovery, but it is tempered by the happenings of the last few years."

"Interesting story! You had a full professional life. How many people can claim to have worked on developing groundbreaking technologies? It had to be rewarding to be

---

[44] I would find out from other sources, not my manager.

part of it, and from the way you talk about it, you also liked mentoring."

"Yes, I did. I loved seeing young engineers finding their true potential. They would tell me I got out of them more than they ever knew they had. That was a joy to experience!"

"What did you learn from your career? What was the gift?"

"Early on I learned that you can achieve whatever you want. It all started with my Master thesis as everyone was telling me I would fail because it was such a new subject, we did not have any literature on it. Going from one scientific paper to the next, writing letters to the authors, tracking down other people interested in the field, and eventually going to another city to build the physical computer[45], produced a thesis that not only got the highest possible mark, but also got me an offer to continue my work through a Ph.D.

I also learned that I had to work in a way that made people forget I was a woman, in a way that broke preconceived ideas. I worked very long hours, readily helped others with my ideas, and, once done with my deliverables, I helped others with theirs. Slowly, they forgot the label 'woman engineer' and I became an 'engineer' like everyone else.

I also learned that to obtain interesting assignments, I needed to deal with the less interesting ones first and prove that I could deliver them on time and within budget. Slowly

---

[45] In Romania, obtaining the necessary parts to build the computer was very difficult, so I went to a university that was willing to provide them.

the assignments would become more and more complex and, as such, more interesting.

As every workplace has its ups and downs, I learned to find joy in the things I liked doing and take the rest as the path to better assignments. This worked every time. People needed complex projects delivered on time.

I also learned that sharing my knowledge would make me a better professional. The questions would challenge my ideas and they would become clearer in my mind.

As far as the gift in all this, how many people can claim having worked on so many interesting projects in their professional life, having met so many talented people, and having helped so many young people start or reinvent their careers? Each of those was a precious gift for me."

"If you could restart your professional life, what would you change about it?" asked Isabelle.

"Nothing, absolutely nothing! Even in the most difficult moments, working with talented engineers who challenged me to do my best was a pleasure. I wish my grandkids could experience as much professional satisfaction as I did. I know they already have two wonderful mentors: their parents."

"Anything else you need to look at before we go back?"

"I don't think so. This was a very fast trip. I 'saw' more than I verbalized, like when the company installed a teletype at my home so I could run computer simulations via the phone line, when I presented at conferences, wrote technical articles, was assigned to a country-wide consortium to develop new technologies, or when I defined a test approach capable of testing all the electronics in a car or truck in only one minute. All these and many more are my 'treasures' and thinking of the people I met on the way fills me with gratitude.

I think I need to take some time now and absorb all this. I never quite saw my career this way, I was too absorbed by the details."

"It sounds like you are ready to come back. Just step through the mirror and walk through your garden, bringing with you the feelings of gratitude and accomplishment for an interesting career. Let me know when you are ready to step through the mirror."

"I am. I am stepping through it right now."

"Look back at all the five mirrors. Do you feel you need additional exploration to determine what is inside any of them?"

"I believe I am done. I am so full of emotions, in part for the recognition of what my life really meant and in part for completing this emotional trip. Walking through my quiet garden I realize I am on a real 'high' from reviewing all those amazing memories. I never really put them together this way. I feel as if I am carrying a substantial gift, that of the realization of the amazing things I have witnessed and the exceptional people I met. I am deeply grateful!"

"When you are ready, open your eyes."

As I opened my eyes I saw Isabelle waiting patiently for me to come back and adjust to the real world.

"Do you think you are done? Is there anything else you need?"

"I believe I am done" I replied. "We achieved what we set out to do. I know now that my life mattered and everything that happened in my life formed the person I am today. I am in your debt for your skillful direction that kept me focused. You were yet another gift for me. Thank you!"

With that, I stood up, we embraced, and I stepped out in the cold winter weather feeling warm and laden with gifts. Yes, I could relax. I knew why and how my life events happened and I owned all its gifts.

Gaining Insight into Being a Professional

Work through this questionnaire for each one of your professions/ jobs. For example, if you worked for several companies, it is interesting to figure out what each one brought into your life. If you have multiple professions, do it for each of them.

As a ……………….. I was……………………………………………………..

…………………………………………………………………………………………..

…………………………………………………………………………………………..

[For example: As a computer design engineer, with XYZ Corporation from….. to…… developing new computer architectures I believe I used my full potential.]

The negative memories I have about my job are:

1 ……………………………………………………………………………
……………………………………………………………………………
……………………………………………………………………………
2. ……………………………………………………………………………
……………………………………………………………………………
……………………………………………………………………………
3. ……………………………………………………………………………
……………………………………………………………………………
……………………………………………………………………………
4. ……………………………………………………………………………
……………………………………………………………………………

....

5. ....

....

....

Because of the negative experiences I had with this job I decided:

1. ....

....

....

2. ....

....

....

3. ....

....

....

4. ....

....

....

5. ....

....

....

[For example: because of the negative experiences I had with this job, I decided to ask more questions about a prospective one, before accepting an offer.]

My positive life decisions as a result of my negative experiences connected with this job are:

1. ....
....
....

2. ....
....
....

3. ....
....
....

4. ....
....
....

5. ....
....
....

[For example: because of the negative experiences with this job I became aware of my strengths as an engineer and, from then on, I looked for jobs that fully took advantage of my strengths.]

The positive memories related to this job are:

1. ....
....
....

2. ....
....
....

3. ....
....

4. ....
....
....
....

5. ....
....
....

Because of the positive experiences I had with this job, I decided to/that:

1. ....
....
....

2. ....
....
....

3. ....
....
....

4. ....
....
....

5. ....
....
....

[For example: because of the positive results I had trying to design with a completely new technology, I decided that stretching my knowledge is fun; I searched for assignments that went beyond my current expertise.]

The top five blessings that come from my experiences with this job, are:

1. ....
....
....

2. ....
....
....

3. ....
....
....

4. ....
....
....

5. ....
....
....

[For example: I learned that I was a much better engineer than I thought I was, which boosted to my self-esteem.]

Acknowledgments
CЗ୫Ͻ

First and foremost, I am deeply grateful to all those I worked with over the years. They taught me about resilience, the value of forgiveness, and how one can literally change one's life by releasing the emotional baggage accumulated over the years. Since many people are shying away from going through therapy, this book intended to give an insight into what happens during therapy sessions.

I would not have attempted to write this book without the encouragement from doctor Paula Jorné, an exceptionally insightful psychotherapist. The tireless encouragement provided by Ann Wagenberg, my friend and mentor, was priceless. I am deeply grateful to Kelly Bruce, Vanessa Rowan, Tina Day, and Tsila Pleasant, who took the time to read the manuscript and give me valuable feedback.

Lucille Halberstadt did an excellent job proofreading the manuscript. She managed to keep my "voice" while correcting the errors and making the book more readable.

Thank you all for helping me birth my book!

About the Author

CƷ℞Ɔ

An inventor, healer, writer, and speaker, Susana Stoica earned a PhD in computer engineering. She practiced her engineering profession on three continents, gaining an appreciation of both the unique and common cultural and healing traditions of people from different parts of the world.

At the peak of her professional career, both as a healer and an engineer, Susana suffered two traumatic brain injuries on the same day. With the help of medical professionals and guided by her previous experience as an energy healer, Susana was able to recover from her many injuries.

Today Susana, in better health than most people of her age, is again living a full life. She is writing, doing her healing work, educating people on how to limit the effects of brain injury, and teaching people how to recover brain function after a concussion or stroke.

Susana has professional training as a Healing Touch

Practitioner, Hypnotherapist, and Journey™ Practitioner, and she is self-taught in many other alternative healing methods. She strives continuously to gain ever-deeper insights into the workings of the human energy system and its relationship with the physical body, and she is consistently amazed and humbled by its complexity and perfect functionality.